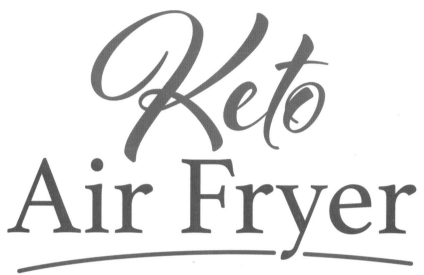

Keto Air Fryer

100+ Delicious Low-Carb Recipes to
Heal Your Body & Help You Lose Weight

INTERNATIONAL BESTSELLING AUTHOR

Maria Emmerich

Victory Belt Publishing Inc
Las Vegas

First published in 2019 by Victory Belt Publishing Inc.

ISBN-13: 978-1-628603-91-0

The author is not a licensed practitioner, physician, or medical professional and offers no medical diagnoses, treatments, suggestions, or counseling. The information presented herein has not been evaluated by the U.S. Food and Drug Administration, and it is not intended to diagnose, treat, cure, or prevent any disease. Full medical clearance from a licensed physician should be obtained before beginning or modifying any diet, exercise, or lifestyle program, and physicians should be informed of all nutritional changes.

The author claims no responsibility to any person or entity for any liability, loss, or damage caused or alleged to be caused directly or indirectly as a result of the use, application, or interpretation of the information presented herein.

Cover design by Crizalie Olimpo
Front and back cover photos by Hayley Mason and Bill Staley
Recipe photos by Maria Emmerich and Jenny Ross
Interior design and illustrations by Yordan Terziev and Boryana Yordanova

Printed in Canada
TC 0119

Contents

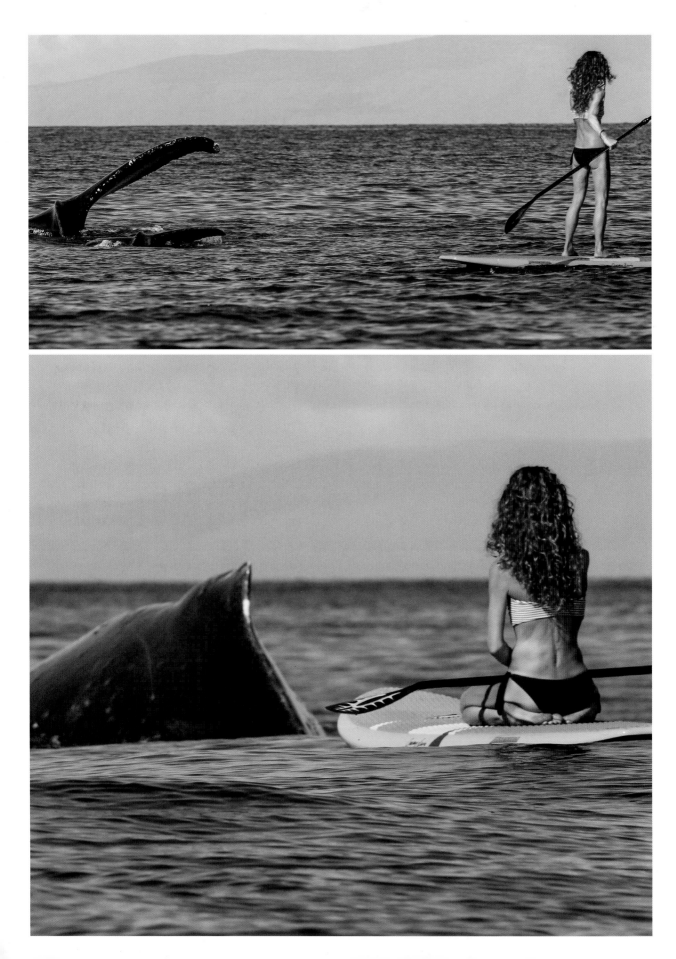

Preface

When I finished my last book, *Keto Instant Pot*, my plan was to take a break and slow down to enjoy some time with my family. My boys are growing up too fast. If I could, I would freeze Micah and Kai at the ages they are at, eight and nine. They are funny, love to play board games every night, and help me in the kitchen.

But I've been told this many times: "If you want to hear God laugh, tell him what you have planned!" And it couldn't be more true in many aspects of my life. Despite my plans for a break, when Erich, my publisher, called to discuss an air fryer book, I couldn't say no. I use my air fryer almost daily, so, to be honest, a keto air fryer book was destined to happen!

Fortunately, I was able to spend time with my boys while creating the recipes for this book. We had so much fun playing in the kitchen and crafting delicious air fryer recipes. Sure, we didn't play as many games of Boggle or Monopoly, but we adapted and had a great time!

It was an especially wonderful time because I had the great pleasure to write this book at the Keto Condo in Maui, which is the condo we own and rent out when we are not there. We call it the Keto Condo because I have all of my favorite keto books on the shelves, and we provide guests with a welcome basket filled with keto goodies. Many times I would write early in the morning before the sun came up, and for a break, I would head out on my paddleboard. Many times I went so far out that I came upon beautiful humpback whales!

My hope is that you get as much enjoyment from making these recipes as I did from creating them. Maybe they'll provide an opportunity for you to spend time with your own children or grandchildren. And whether you're cooking in Maui or Minnesota or Miami, I hope you find pleasure every day in living and eating healthy.

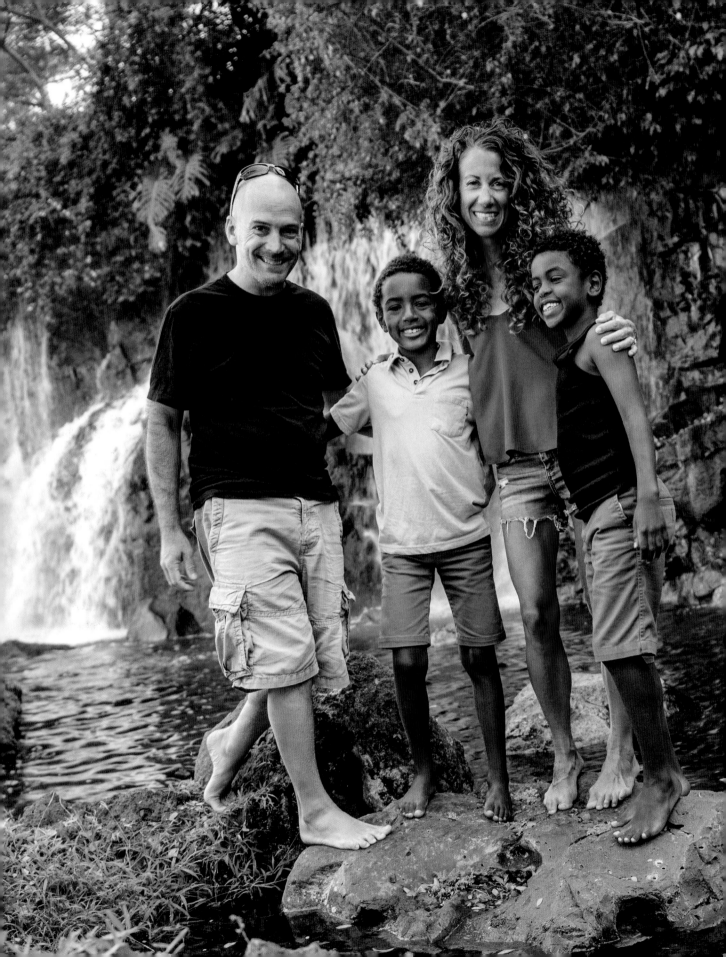

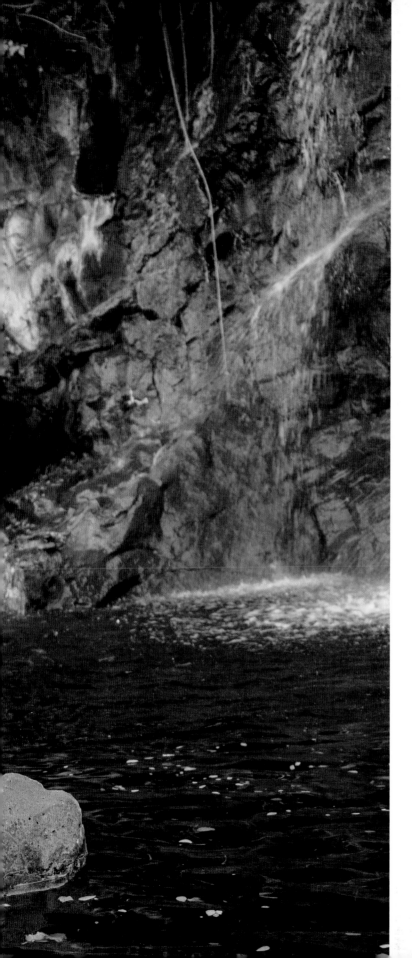

Note to Readers

Like many of you, I have had some really difficult times in my life. Life is like ocean waves, constantly rising and falling; everyone has high points as well as low points. It was during a low point that I had to stop spending money at restaurants and start cooking at home, and that ultimately helped me become the healthy ketogenic cook I am today. I have learned to accept the lows and have gratitude for the highs. The hardships I've experienced taught me amazing lifelong lessons. I struggled out of the cocoon, and that struggle made me a butterfly with strong wings.

I want to dedicate this book to you—yes, you. It is you and your support that have made my life possible. About four months after we adopted our baby boys, many years ago, my husband, Craig, lost his job. We kept this secret for a long time. It was such a scary time for us, and Craig didn't want to feel like he was failing his family. But thanks to all of you, my boys have the best stay-at-home dad ever! It is because of all of your support that we have our family.

Thank you, thank you, thank you, from all of us—Maria, Craig, Micah, and Kai!

Keto Basics

You may have heard that a ketogenic diet is high in fat, moderate in protein, and low in carbs. But while there is more to a well-formulated ketogenic diet, there is really only one requirement to become ketogenic, and that is to cut your dietary carbs low enough.

Becoming ketogenic is about changing your body's primary fuel from glucose—which all carbohydrates break down into—to fat. It takes some time for the body to become efficient at using fat, but when it is, you're "fat adapted" or "keto adapted."

When the body is keto adapted, it primarily uses fat (free fatty acids, or FFA) as its fuel. Some of this FFA goes to the liver and is turned into ketones to fuel parts of the body that can only run on glucose or ketones, like parts of the brain. It turns out that the brain loves running on ketones, and you get better moods, mental clarity, and more as a result. About 60 to 70 percent of the brain can run on ketones, and the brain thrives when it does as the brain prefers to run on ketones. Being ketogenic also has a wide range of health benefits, and it's often accompanied by a drop in body fat.

But higher blood ketones is not associated with better results. Blood ketones are just the difference in fuel generated and fuel used. Also, the longer you are keto adapted the lower your blood ketones will be as your body is more efficient at using them. So don't worry about trying to get higher blood ketones. You could be 0.4 mmol/L and have great results.

There are many ways to become ketogenic, some healthy and some not so healthy. Here are just some of them:

- Keep dietary carbs low (below 30 grams per day or so).

- Get 90 percent of your calories from fat.

- Eat no fat while keeping carbs very low.

- Eat lots of trans fats and vegetable oils while keeping carbs low.

- Don't eat anything for a period of time; exactly how long depends on your age (see the chart at right). Infants are always ketogenic—their blood ketone levels range from 0.5 mmol/L in a fed state to 2.0 mmol/L about two hours after eating—but it generally takes adults longer.

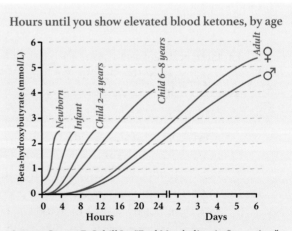

Hours until you show elevated blood ketones, by age

Source: George F. Cahill Jr., "Fuel Metabolism in Starvation," *Annual Review of Nutrition* 26 (2006): 1–22.

During fasting, the body uses fat for fuel, which raises ketone levels. The younger the individual, the faster ketone levels rise—but everyone becomes ketogenic eventually.

As you can see, some methods for becoming ketogenic are obviously not very healthy (eating trans fats, for instance—they may help you become ketogenic, but they're associated with heart disease, stroke, and type 2 diabetes).

So what exactly does a genuinely healthy, well-formulated ketogenic diet look like? How do you know if you're eating the right proportion of macronutrients? Let's look at carb, protein, and fat in turn and talk about what to track for each, and then look at what a well-formulated ketogenic diet looks like overall.

Carb

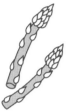

The most important part of keto is getting your carb intake right. For most people, consuming fewer than 30 grams of total carbs a day is the best way to switch to burning fat instead of glucose.

However, your carbohydrate tolerance depends on a lot of factors. Some athletes can eat up to 50 grams or so a day and stay in ketosis because they are very active. On the other hand, people with metabolic issues, such as type 2 diabetes, need to stay under 20 grams a day.

You may have heard of "net carbs," which is the total amount of carbs you consume minus the amount of fiber. But some kinds of fiber, such as inulin, can affect blood sugar, so I recommend always counting total carbs and then subtracting any carbs that come from erythritol, a noncaloric sweetener that isn't digested and therefore doesn't affect blood sugar. The nutritional information for all my recipes shows the amount of carbs with erythritol carbs already subtracted.

Protein

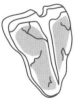

Getting the right amount of protein should be your second priority, right after limiting your carb intake. Protein builds and repairs lean mass (muscles, soft tissues, and many other critical body parts), and as we age, sustaining lean mass is crucial for vitality and longevity.

To find your protein goal, multiply your lean body mass (your total weight minus your body fat) by 0.8. For example, if you weigh 180 pounds and have 40 percent body fat, you have 108 pounds of lean mass. So your protein goal would be 86 grams of protein a day (0.8 x 108). You can either hit this goal every day or average it out over the course of a week, so that by week's end you've consumed the same amount of protein as if you ate the optimal amount every day. This ensures that you maintain your muscle and lean mass.

If you are trying to gain muscle, you can go higher in protein, 0.9 or 1.0 times your lean mass. And as we age, we need even more protein just to maintain our lean mass. If you're over sixty, you should consume 1.0 to 1.5 times your lean mass. And if you have a chronic disease, aim for 1.5 times your lean mass.

Kids need even more protein to support their growth and development. Infants need about 3.0 times their lean mass in protein grams per day. Children ages four to thirteen need about 2.0 times their lean mass. Teens need about 1.5 times their lean mass or more, until they stop growing.

Fat

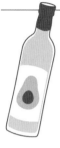

Fat intake is the last piece of the macros puzzle. Once you've figured out your carb limit and protein goal, you can adjust your fat intake based on your overall goals.

When you are keto adapted, your body can use body fat and dietary fat equally. The more dietary fat you consume, the less stored body fat is used for fuel. So if weight loss is your goal, consuming less fat will help use more stored body fat as fuel. When you are closer to your goal weight, you can add more fat to find your body's maintenance point.

A good rule of thumb for weight loss is to make your target grams of fat the same as or less than your target grams of protein. During your first couple of weeks on keto, you may want to eat more fat than that to help with hunger and cravings. But as soon as cravings diminish and hunger reduces, dial your fat intake down so that you can burn more body fat and thus lose weight faster.

Calculating Macros

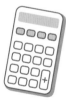

With the guidelines above in mind, here's an example of how you can calculate your own macros. Let's look at a woman who is forty-five years old, weighs 180 pounds, and is five feet three inches tall. She has 40 percent body fat and some degree of metabolic syndrome (such as insulin resistance and high blood pressure), and she wants to lose weight.

Because she has some metabolic issues, she would eat no more than 20 grams total carbs per day, and with her amount of lean body mass, her protein goal would be about 86 grams per day. Since she wants to lose weight, her fat target is the same as her protein target, 86 grams per day, or less (though she might exceed that in the first couple of weeks to manage cravings and hunger).

Nutrient Density

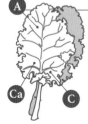

As important as your macros are, micronutrients are just as important. You can eat a diet that falls right in line with your macros, but if your carbs, protein, and fat aren't coming from nutritious sources, you won't be giving your body what it needs to be healthy. Plus, consuming foods devoid of nutrients means that you don't get the "I'm full" signal as quickly as you do with nutrient-dense foods.

So what are some of the most nutrient-dense foods? Let's take a look at some of the most popular "superfoods" and beef.

Nutrients in "superfoods" compared to animal protein

Per serving	Apples	Blue-berries	Kale	Beef	Beef Liver
Calcium (mg)	9.1	4.5	63.4	11.0	11.0
Magnesium (mg)	7.3	4.5	15.0	19.0	18.0
Phosphorus (mg)	20.0	9.0	24.6	175.0	387.0
Potassium (mg)	163.8	57.8	200.6	370.0	380.0
Iron (mg)	0.2	0.2	0.8	3.3	8.8
Zinc (mg)	0.2	0.2	0.2	4.5	4.0
Selenium (mcg)	0.0	0.1	0.4	14.2	39.7
Vitamin A (IU)	69.2	40.5	13530.9	40.0	53400.0
Vitamin B6 (mg)	0.0	0.1	0.1	0.4	1.1
Vitamin B12 (mcg)	0.0	0.0	0.1	2.0	11.0
Vitamin C (mg)	7.3	7.3	36.1	2.0	27.0
Vitamin D (IU)	0.0	0.0	0.0	7.0	19.0
Vitamin E (mg)	0.2	0.5	0.8	1.7	0.6
Niacin (mg)	0.2	0.3	0.4	4.8	17.0
Folate (mcg)	0.0	4.5	11.4	6.0	145.0

Nutrients in butter coffee compared to white bread and animal protein

Per 400 calories	Butter Coffee	White Bread	Eggs	Beef
Calcium (mg)	6.8	65.9	132.0	23.5
Magnesium (mg)	0.6	0.0	26.4	40.7
Phosphorus (mg)	6.8	0.0	454.0	374.5
Potassium (mg)	6.8	0.0	332.0	791.8
Iron (mg)	0.0	4.8	3.1	7.1
Zinc (mg)	0.0	0.0	2.8	9.6
Selenium (mcg)	0.3	0.0	81.3	30.4
Vitamin A (IU)	709.0	0.0	1372.8	85.6
Vitamin B6 (mg)	0.0	0.0	0.3	0.9
Vitamin B12 (mcg)	0.0	0.0	2.9	4.3
Vitamin C (mg)	0.0	0.0	0.0	4.3
Vitamin D (IU)	2.9	0.0	229.7	15.0
Vitamin E (mg)	0.7	0.0	2.7	3.6
Niacin (mg)	0.0	0.0	0.2	10.3
Folate (mcg)	0.9	0.0	116.2	12.8
Protein	0.2	13.0	33.0	77.0

The most nutrient-dense food isn't kale or blueberries or apples; it's beef liver! That's right, both beef and beef liver have more nutrients across a wider range of vitamins and minerals than any fruit or vegetable.

Let's take this one step further and look at the nutrient density of butter coffee. Butter coffee is commonly recommended in the keto community by people who say keto is about adding lots of fat to the diet. The chart below compares butter coffee (made with MCT oil, butter, and cream) with white bread, eggs, and beef, and it shows why butter coffee isn't the healthiest option.

Like processed foods, butter coffee is high in calories and very low in most vitamins and minerals. I am not saying butter coffee is the same as processed foods—MCT oil, butter, and cream are all healthy sources of fats. But if weight loss is your goal, you want your body using stored body fat for fuel, not dietary fat. And even if weight loss isn't the goal, it is always better to choose whole foods that come with a lot more vitamins and minerals instead of adding fat just to increase your fat intake.

Air Fryer 101

Air fryers are becoming more and more popular, and for good reason! They are fantastic for making healthy, delicious meals in no time. An air fryer is basically a very high-powered convection oven that uses heated circulating air to cook foods in a unique way that resembles frying without the large amounts of oil. No mess, no grease!

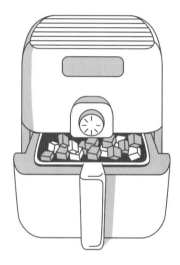

Plus, air fryers do a lot more than fry. You can use an air fryer to grill and roast meats, bake desserts, even hard-boil eggs! I love to use it to reheat leftovers, too.

Why Use an Air Fryer on Keto?

You may be thinking, *Air fryer? I thought keto was high-fat. Why not use a deep fryer?*

True, deep fryers use a lot of oil, which has high amounts of fat. And as long as you're using stable, healthy oils, like avocado oil (and never processed vegetable oils), some deep-fried foods are fine.

But it's a common misconception that you need to eat a ton of fat on keto. If your body is already "high fat," your diet doesn't need to be.

Imagine a bucket of water with a valve on the bottom. If you add more water to the bucket with the valve open, the water level doesn't rise—and if the valve is open enough, it even drops. But if the valve is shut, the water level rises.

This is what happens with fat-burning in your body. If you're consuming more dietary fat, you need to be burning the same amount of fat—the valve needs to be wide open—or the level of fat in your body rises.

This is something of an oversimplification, of course, because there are a lot of other factors at play when it comes to fat storage and weight loss. But it gives you an idea of why simply eating a ton of fat isn't the healthiest way to be keto.

Top Ten Reasons to Love Your Air Fryer

1. Best way to reheat leftovers
Ever pop a slice of keto pizza in the microwave to reheat it and get back a soggy mess? The air fryer is a perfect solution: it reheats quickly and easily and keeps a nice crisp on baked and fried foods.

2. Makes crispy veggies in no time
If you love lightly charred veggies, as I do, an air fryer is perfect: veggies come out nicely caramelized. My favorite is air-fried Brussels sprouts—so good!

3. Makes the juiciest hamburgers in an instant
I love hamburgers and prefer to have one every day. To make an easy family dinner, all I have to do is shape ground meat into patties, season them with my keto burger seasoning, and toss them in the air fryer. Tip of the day: Salt draws out moisture, so don't season the meat until right before you cook the burgers, so they stay nice and moist.

4. Makes amazing bacon without a mess
My son likes his bacon chewy whereas I like mine crispy. I remove his about 90 seconds before mine, and they both come out perfect!

5. Doesn't heat up the house on hot summer days
My husband often jokes that I'd turn my oven on to make keto bread when it is 99°F out. It's true, but now I use my air fryer, which doesn't heat up the house. We can even use it in Maui at the Keto Condo!

6. Saves time
The cool thing about an air fryer is that it takes just a fraction of the time to preheat that an oven does—and you don't have to preheat at all if you don't want to. That means even less time in the kitchen, and you save on energy costs.

7. Makes delicious steaks that are crispy on the outside, juicy on the inside
Enough said!

8. Easy cleanup
I used to fry dishes in a cast-iron skillet with oil, and the cleanup was a hassle. I had oil splatters everywhere, including my hood range, which was impossible to clean. Plus, the smell of deep frying filled my house for days. With air frying, there is really no mess to clean up, and no smell!

9. Fun for kids
My son loves to make bacon and English muffin pizzas in the air fryer, and he can do it without my help! Kids can easily cook with an air fryer. It's a great tool to help get them interested in making homemade meals.

10. Great for camping!
As long as you have a campsite with electricity, you can use your air fryer when you go camping. When we go RV camping, I take our air fryer, and it makes meals in an instant.

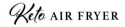

Using an Air Fryer Instead of the Oven

Just about every recipe that uses an oven can be made in an air fryer, with a few changes. Adjusting the temperatures of your favorite recipes takes a little time and practice, but most often you will have to lower the air fryer temperature. For example, I find that when I make my biscuits in the oven, it needs to be set to 400°F, but when I make them in the air fryer, it has to be only 350°F or the biscuits burn. I recommend starting by lowering the temperature around 25°F from the oven setting, and don't leave the food in the air fryer as long.

Once you figure out the best temperature for cooking recipes in an air fryer instead of the oven, it works really well. That said, there's one exception I have to mention: I'm not a huge fan of making cheesecakes in my air fryer. Since air frying involves pushing around heated air, it causes lots of cracking in cheesecakes—the fans dry out the top of the cheesecake. In fact, anything that contains a lot of eggs needs to stay moist on top while the interior is still rising and setting; otherwise, you will get the infamous cheesecake crack on top. An air fryer isn't the best choice for these foods.

Maria's Air Fryer Tips

1. Invest in a larger air fryer. When I had a smaller air fryer, only 2.75 quarts, I was frustrated at how little the basket was. It was fine for cooking for one person, but if you're cooking for a family or like to have leftovers for an easy keto meal after a long day of work, you'll want something larger. My favorite is a combination toaster oven–air fryer (see box), but you can also get larger air fryers that are 4 to 6 quarts.

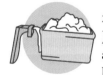

2. Don't overcrowd the basket. Just another reason to get a larger air fryer! If you overstuff the basket, there will be spots on the food where the air can't circulate; these spots will stay cold and/or uncooked. Don't be tempted to try to fit more food in the basket than fits easily. If you have a smaller air fryer and the recipe makes too much to fit in the basket, work in batches and you'll get a much better end result.

3. Invest in a spray bottle just for oil. I always use a spray bottle with a pump to mist my air fryer basket and foods with oil to avoid sticking. I fill my spray bottle with avocado oil because it's a healthy, stable oil that can handle high temperatures. Avoid aerosol oil sprays, which can ruin the basket lining.

The Air Fryer I Recommend
Personally, I love the Cuisinart TOA-60, which is a combination air fryer and toaster oven. It is much larger than most air fryers—the interior is 0.6 cubic feet—but it isn't heavy (I can move it from my pantry to kitchen with ease). Cuisinart doesn't pay me to mention them, but I adore Cuisinart customer service. When my Cuisinart ice cream maker died because of overuse (I had it for seven years and used it weekly), they sent me a new one for free!

4. Flip food halfway through cooking.

Just as with a traditional oven, most foods need to be flipped halfway through to ensure even cooking.

5. Invest in oven-safe gloves.

When you're trying to flip those foods halfway through cooking, sometimes you just have to use your hands. I highly suggest investing in a good pair of oven-safe gloves. They're inexpensive, and they come in handy with other kinds of cooking, too, not just the air fryer.

6. Wipe up grease to avoid white smoke.

Often when you air fry foods with a high fat content, such as bacon or chicken wings, grease can splatter and hit the heating element, and the result is white smoke rising from the fryer. Don't fret, it doesn't harm your food or the air fryer, but it is bothersome. When it happens, just stop the air fryer, take out the food and remove the basket, and dab the grease with paper towels to soak up the oil. Then start the cooking process again.

7. Reheat food in the air fryer instead of the microwave.

Food that's been reheated in the microwave never is as crispy and delicious as when you first made it. Reheating leftovers in the air fryer is safe and creates a delicious, crispy outside, just like when the food was freshly made.

8. Adapt recipes written for a traditional oven.

When you're using an air fryer with a recipe that's written for a traditional oven, you'll often need to reduce the temperature and cooking time. For example, my biscuits for Valerie's Breakfast Sammies (page 34) would be cooked at 400°F in an oven, but in the air fryer, that temperature would scorch the heck out of these delicious biscuits. For best results, adapt a recipe written for a traditional oven by lowering the temperature around 25°F and don't leave the food in the air fryer as long.

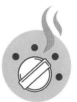

9. Get in the habit of preheating.

You don't always have to preheat your air fryer, and many recipes don't mention doing this, but it helps ensure even cooking.

10. Use a baking pan.

Most air fryers come with baking pans, but if yours didn't, I highly suggest getting one or two 6 by 3-inch pans to make dishes such as my Denver Omelet (page 30).

Cooked Internal Temperatures

Rare	125°F
Medium-rare	135°F
Medium	145°F
Medium-well	155°F
Well-done	165°F

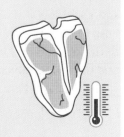

Got 10 Minutes? Make a Home-Cooked Meal!

These quick and easy recipes are cooked in just ten minutes with your air fryer—faster than takeout!

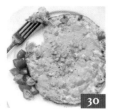 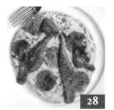 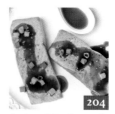 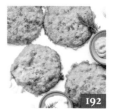 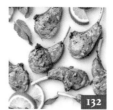

Denver Omelet 30   **Breakfast Pizza** 28   **Mojito Lamb Chops** 132   **Asian Marinated Salmon** 204   **Tuna Melt Croquettes** 192

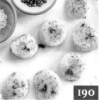 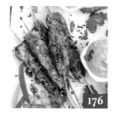 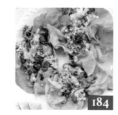 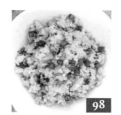

Simple Scallops 190   **Chicken Strips with Satay Sauce** 176   **Thai Tacos with Peanut Sauce** 184   **Fried Cauliflower Rice** 98

Make-Ahead Recipes for Easy Meals

These recipes all freeze and reheat well, making them perfect for make-ahead meals—on a busy weeknight, all you have to do is heat them up and eat! They're great for leftovers, too.

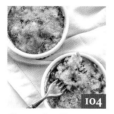 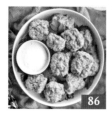 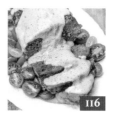 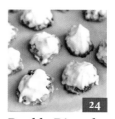 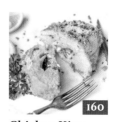

Crunchy-Top Personal Mac 'n' Cheese 104   **Keto Tots** 86   **Swedish Meatloaf** 116   **Double-Dipped Mini Cinnamon Biscuits** 24   **Chicken Kiev** 160

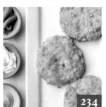 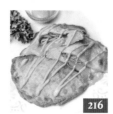 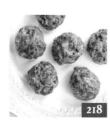 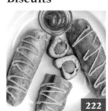 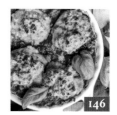

Chicken Patties 234   **Ham 'n' Cheese Hand Pies** 216   **Cheeseburger Meatballs** 218   **No-Corn Dogs** 222   **Mama Maria's Savory Sausage Cobbler** 146

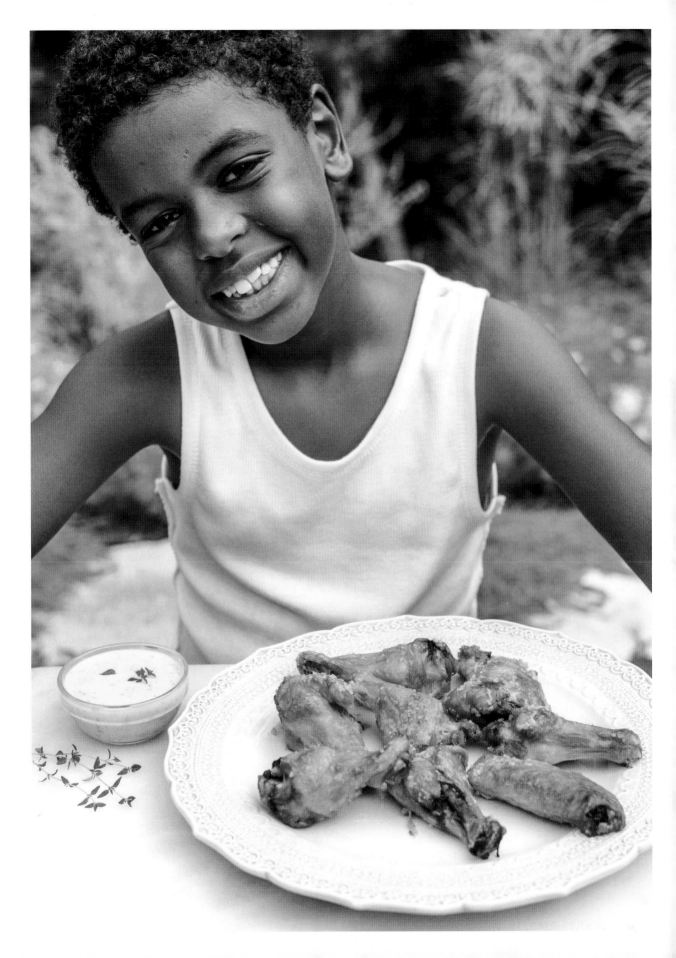

Ingredient Tips

My recipes use ordinary, everyday ingredients that you can find at any grocery store—but if you're new to keto cooking, it may be helpful to learn a little more about keto-friendly ingredients.

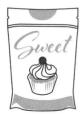

Sweeteners

I always recommend using keto-friendly sweeteners that don't affect blood sugar. This means avoiding table sugar, honey, maple syrup, and other traditional sweeteners. But that doesn't mean you have to use artificial sweeteners! Erythritol, my favorite sweetener, is all natural—it's found in certain fruits and root vegetables—and doesn't affect blood sugar.

In my recipes, I prefer to use Swerve brand confectioners'-style sweetener, which is made primarily of erythritol. Swerve is available in granular and powdered form, but I find that the powdered (confectioners') form results in a smoother finished product. If you're using a granular form of erythritol, such as Wholesome! All-Natural Zero, you can pulverize it in a blender or coffee grinder to get the powdered texture.

If a recipe specifically calls for powdered or liquid sweetener, do not substitute any other sweetener. These recipes rely on these particular sweeteners—for example, some sweeteners won't work in recipes where the sweetener has to melt—so it's important to use exactly what's called for.

If a sweetener in an ingredients list is followed by "or equivalent," such as "¼ cup Swerve confectioners'-style sweetener or equivalent amount of liquid or powdered sweetener," you are free to use any keto-friendly sweetener, liquid or powdered. For example, you could use liquid stevia, stevia glycerite, monk fruit, Zsweet, or xylitol.

I've used Swerve, my favorite keto-friendly sweetener, in many of the recipes in this book. But if you prefer to use another keto-friendly sweetener, here are the conversion ratios:

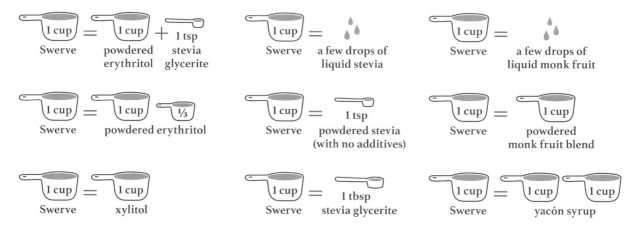

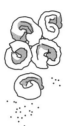

Pork Dust

Pork dust—pork rinds ground into a fine powder, also called pork panko—makes a great zero-carb breading that gives air fryer recipes a crispy crust. You can find pastured pork rinds at most stores. I've even found them at airports! For breading, my favorite kind is Pork Cloud brand garlic thyme pork rinds. But feel free to use any flavor in my recipes!

To make pork dust from pork rinds, place a few handfuls of pork rinds in a high-powered blender or food processor and pulse until you have finely ground pork dust.

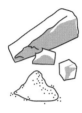

Powdered Parmesan

Some of the recipes in this book call for powdered Parmesan cheese. You can use store-bought Parmesan (called "grated" rather than "powdered"), but I like to make my own. The shreds need to be smaller than grated, so I shred a large block of Parmesan and then pulse the shreds in a food processor until they're very fine. Powdered Parmesan works great for making low-carb breading for crispy chicken, such as my Popcorn Chicken (page 230).

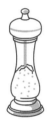

Salts

I jokingly call myself a salt snob. I really like quality salt, so much that I even pack it in my carry-on when I travel, which always causes issues with the TSA. (At the Paris airport, though, when they asked what it was and I told them it was a fancy salt, they smiled and said, "Oh, no problem!") Salt may seem like a minor ingredient in your cooking, but once you start using a quality salt filled with minerals, you will notice a difference in the flavor of your food. Even though it is used in small amounts, salt can take your cooking to the next level!

Redmond Real Salt is from central Utah, where it was deposited by an ancient sea. I always use Redmond salt for a few reasons. First, many times salt has added anticaking agents, such as dextrose, which is a kind of sugar—Redmond doesn't. Second, it has over sixty naturally occurring trace minerals. Finally, it has no microplastics, additives, or chemicals.

Smoked salts are especially good for adding flavor to vegetarian dishes. You can find smoked salts online or in specialty grocery stores.

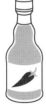

Hot Sauce

When a recipe like my Buffalo Chicken Drumsticks (page 164) calls for hot sauce, I like to use Frank's RedHot. It has no added sugar and no harmful vegetable oils.

Tomato Sauce

When choosing a tomato sauce, always choose an organic one that comes in a glass jar.

Nutrition Data in the Recipes
Each recipe lists the calories and amounts of fat, protein, and carbs in the dish.
Garnishes, optional items, and "for serving" items are not included in this information.

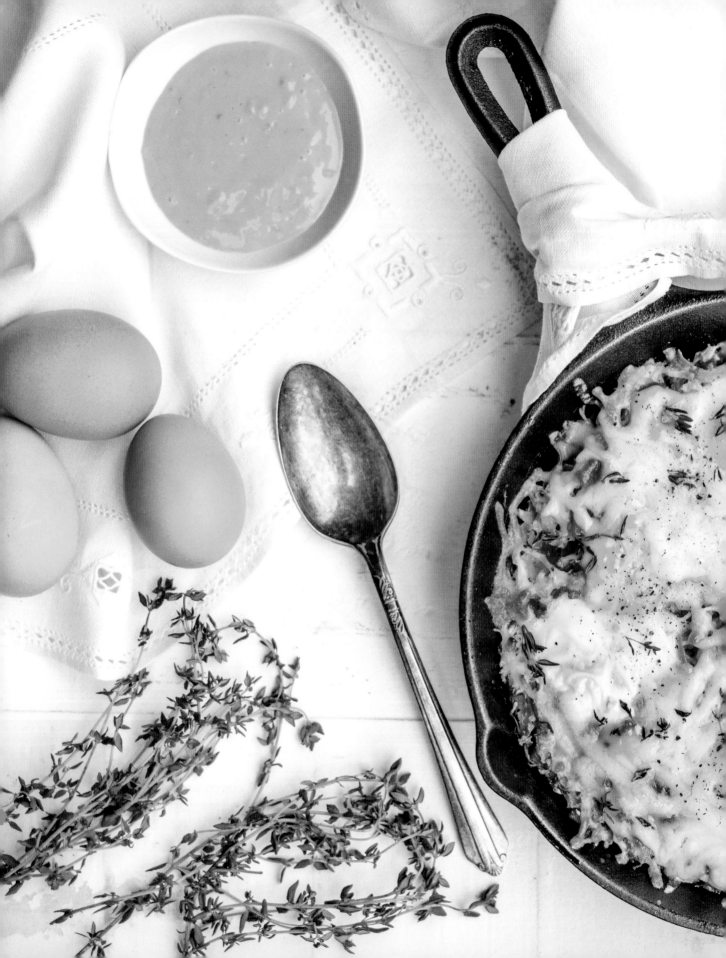

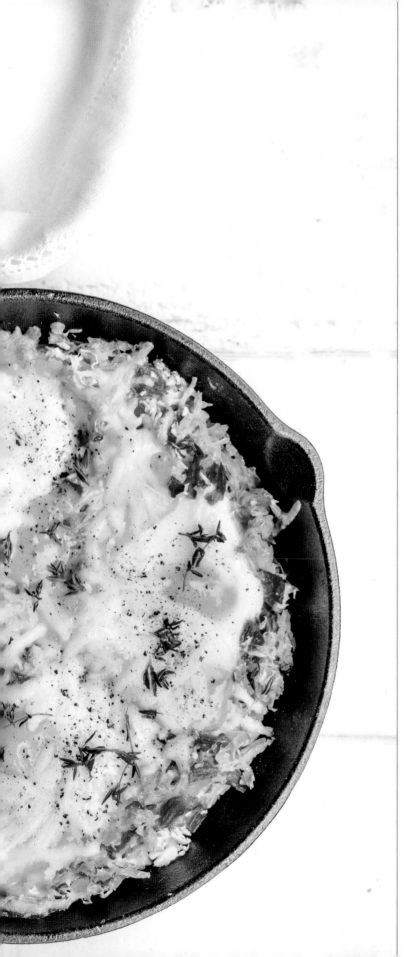

Breakfast

Bacon-and-Eggs Avocado

yield: 1 serving   *prep time:* 5 minutes   *cook time:* 17 minutes

1 large egg

1 avocado, halved, peeled, and pitted

2 slices bacon

Fresh parsley, for serving (optional)

Sea salt flakes, for garnish (optional)

1. Spray the air fryer basket with avocado oil. Preheat the air fryer to 320°F. Fill a small bowl with cool water.

2. Soft-boil the egg: Place the egg in the air fryer basket. Cook for 6 minutes for a soft yolk or 7 minutes for a cooked yolk. Transfer the egg to the bowl of cool water and let sit for 2 minutes. Peel and set aside.

3. Use a spoon to carve out extra space in the center of the avocado halves until the cavities are big enough to fit the soft-boiled egg. Place the soft-boiled egg in the center of one half of the avocado and replace the other half of the avocado on top, so the avocado appears whole on the outside.

4. Starting at one end of the avocado, wrap the bacon around the avocado to completely cover it. Use toothpicks to hold the bacon in place.

5. Place the bacon-wrapped avocado in the air fryer basket and cook for 5 minutes. Flip the avocado over and cook for another 5 minutes, or until the bacon is cooked to your liking. Serve on a bed of fresh parsley, if desired, and sprinkle with salt flakes, if desired.

6. Best served fresh. Store extras in an airtight container in the fridge for up to 4 days. Reheat in a preheated 320°F air fryer for 4 minutes, or until heated through.

note: The keto meter at the top of each recipe indicates where the recipe ranks on the keto "scale": low, medium, or high. Note that in a few cases, a dish's ranking may vary depending on whether you include an optional ingredient or component, such as a sauce.

(per serving)   calories **536** | fat **46g** | protein **18g** | total carbs **18g** | fiber **14g**

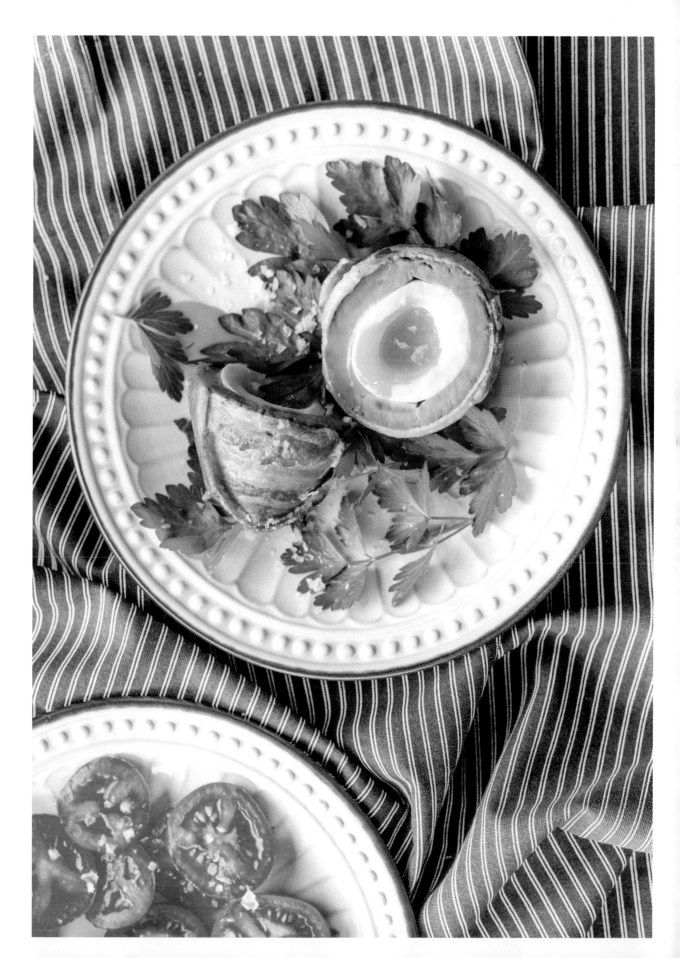

Double-Dipped Mini Cinnamon Biscuits

yield: 8 biscuits (2 per serving) *prep time:* 15 minutes *cook time:* 13 minutes

KETO

2 cups blanched almond flour

½ cup Swerve confectioners'-style sweetener or equivalent amount of liquid or powdered sweetener (see page 18)

1 teaspoon baking powder

½ teaspoon fine sea salt

¼ cup plus 2 tablespoons (¾ stick) very cold unsalted butter

¼ cup unsweetened, unflavored almond milk

1 large egg

1 teaspoon vanilla extract

3 teaspoons ground cinnamon

GLAZE:

½ cup Swerve confectioners'-style sweetener or equivalent amount of powdered sweetener (see page 18)

¼ cup heavy cream or unsweetened, unflavored almond milk

1. Preheat the air fryer to 350°F. Line a pie pan that fits into your air fryer with parchment paper.

2. In a medium-sized bowl, mix together the almond flour, sweetener (if powdered; do not add liquid sweetener), baking powder, and salt. Cut the butter into ½-inch squares, then use a hand mixer to work the butter into the dry ingredients. When you are done, the mixture should still have chunks of butter.

3. In a small bowl, whisk together the almond milk, egg, and vanilla extract (if using liquid sweetener, add it as well) until blended. Using a fork, stir the wet ingredients into the dry ingredients until large clumps form. Add the cinnamon and use your hands to swirl it into the dough.

4. Form the dough into sixteen 1-inch balls and place them on the prepared pan, spacing them about ½ inch apart. (If you're using a smaller air fryer, work in batches if necessary.) Bake in the air fryer until golden, 10 to 13 minutes. Remove from the air fryer and let cool on the pan for at least 5 minutes.

5. While the biscuits bake, make the glaze: Place the powdered sweetener in a small bowl and slowly stir in the heavy cream with a fork.

6. When the biscuits have cooled somewhat, dip the tops into the glaze, allow it to dry a bit, and then dip again for a thick glaze.

7. Serve warm or at room temperature. Store unglazed biscuits in an airtight container in the refrigerator for up to 3 days or in the freezer for up to a month. Reheat in a preheated 350°F air fryer for 5 minutes, or until warmed through, and dip in the glaze as instructed above.

note: When I was a little girl, I always wished cinnamon rolls had more glaze, so these are double-dipped for extra goodness!

(per serving) calories **546** | fat **51g** | protein **14g** | total carbs **13g** | fiber **6g**

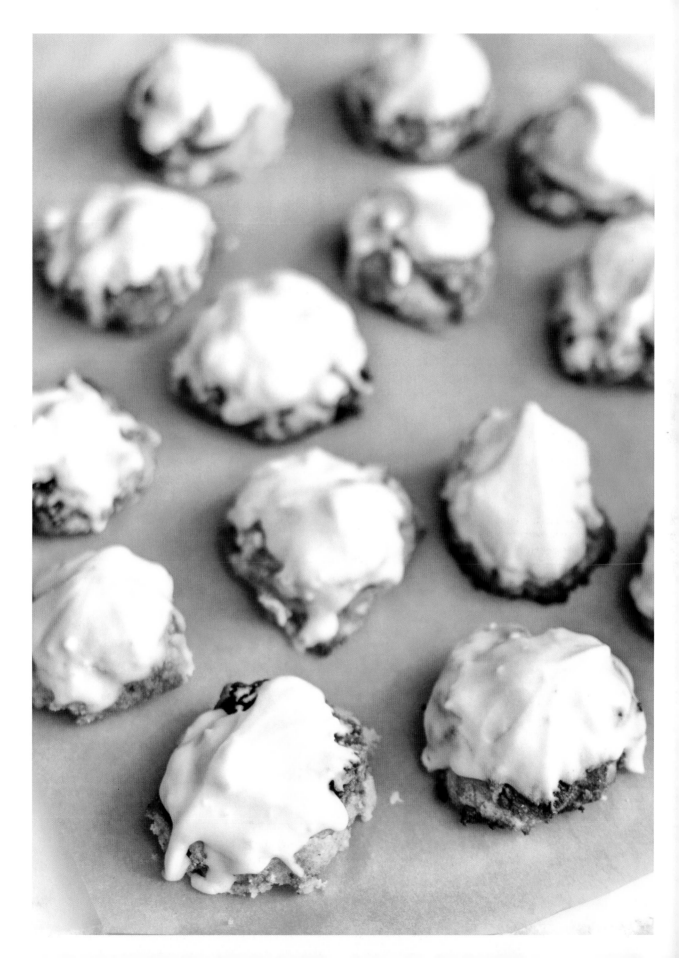

Meritage Eggs

yield: 2 servings   *prep time:* 5 minutes   *cook time:* 8 minutes

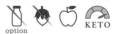

2 teaspoons unsalted butter (or coconut oil for dairy-free), for greasing the ramekins

4 large eggs

2 teaspoons chopped fresh thyme

½ teaspoon fine sea salt

¼ teaspoon ground black pepper

2 tablespoons heavy cream (or unsweetened, unflavored almond milk for dairy-free)

3 tablespoons finely grated Parmesan cheese (or Kite Hill brand chive cream cheese style spread, softened, for dairy-free)

Fresh thyme leaves, for garnish (optional)

1. Preheat the air fryer to 400°F. Grease two 4-ounce ramekins with the butter.

2. Crack 2 eggs into each ramekin and divide the thyme, salt, and pepper between the ramekins. Pour 1 tablespoon of the heavy cream into each ramekin. Sprinkle each ramekin with 1½ tablespoons of the Parmesan cheese.

3. Place the ramekins in the air fryer and cook for 8 minutes for soft-cooked yolks (longer if you desire a harder yolk).

4. Garnish with a sprinkle of ground black pepper and thyme leaves, if desired. Best served fresh.

notes: This recipe is named for Meritage, a lovely restaurant in St. Paul, Minnesota, that serves the most delicious eggs en cocotte.

One of my recipe testers tried using unsweetened almond milk in place of the heavy cream, and used Kite Hill brand dairy-free chive cream cheese style spread in place of the cheese, and the eggs were just as delicious!

(per serving)   calories **331** | fat **29g** | protein **16g** | total carbs **2g** | fiber **0.2g**

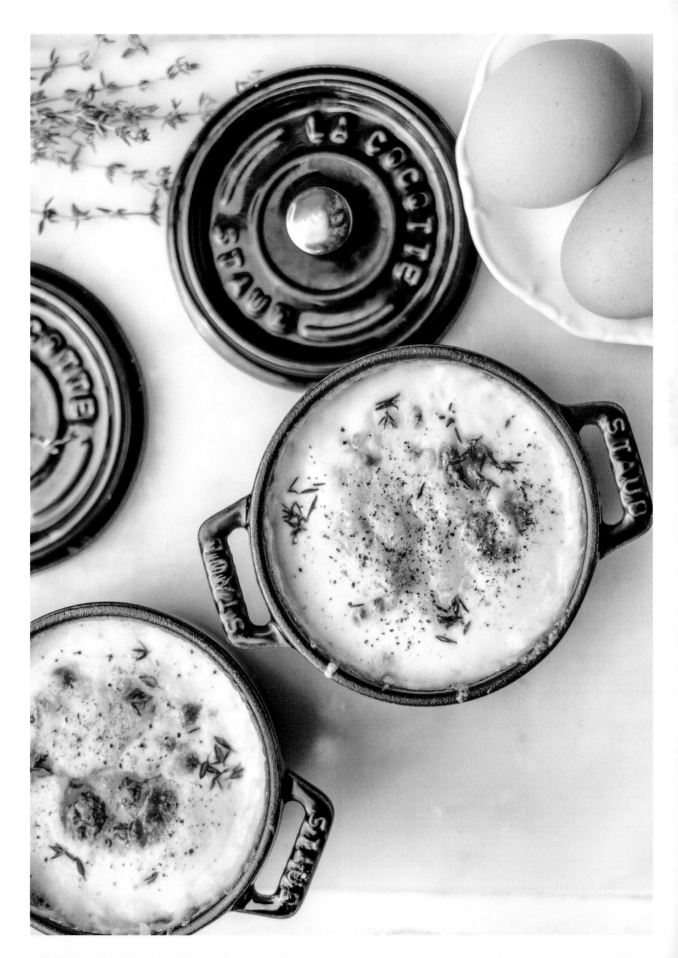

Breakfast Pizza

yield: 1 serving *prep time:* 5 minutes *cook time:* 8 minutes

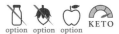
option option option KETO

2 large eggs

¼ cup unsweetened, unflavored almond milk (or unflavored hemp milk for nut-free)

¼ teaspoon fine sea salt

⅛ teaspoon ground black pepper

¼ cup diced onions

¼ cup shredded Parmesan cheese (omit for dairy-free)

6 pepperoni slices (omit for vegetarian)

¼ teaspoon dried oregano leaves

¼ cup pizza sauce, warmed, for serving

1. Preheat the air fryer to 350°F. Grease a 6 by 3-inch cake pan.

2. In a small bowl, use a fork to whisk together the eggs, almond milk, salt, and pepper. Add the onions and stir to mix. Pour the mixture into the greased pan. Top with the cheese (if using), pepperoni slices (if using), and oregano.

3. Place the pan in the air fryer and cook for 8 minutes, or until the eggs are cooked to your liking.

4. Loosen the eggs from the sides of the pan with a spatula and place them on a serving plate. Drizzle the pizza sauce on top. Best served fresh.

(per serving) calories **357** | fat **25g** | protein **24g** | total carbs **9g** | fiber **2g**

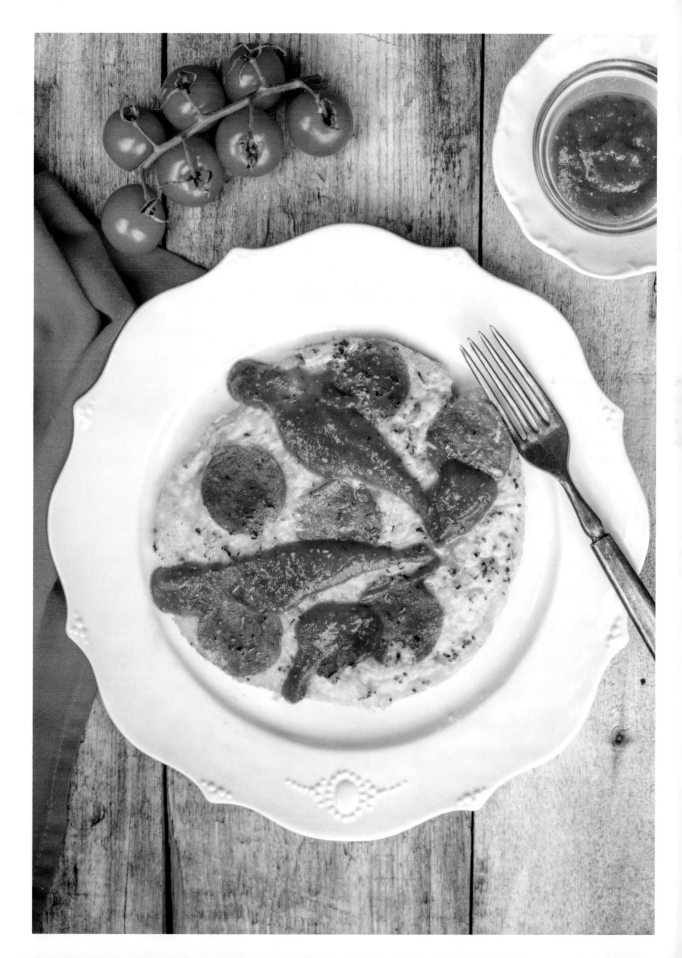

Denver Omelet

yield: 1 serving   *prep time:* 5 minutes   *cook time:* 8 minutes

2 large eggs

¼ cup unsweetened, unflavored almond milk

¼ teaspoon fine sea salt

⅛ teaspoon ground black pepper

¼ cup diced ham (omit for vegetarian)

¼ cup diced green and red bell peppers

2 tablespoons diced green onions, plus more for garnish

¼ cup shredded cheddar cheese (about 1 ounce) (omit for dairy-free)

Quartered cherry tomatoes, for serving (optional)

1. Preheat the air fryer to 350°F. Grease a 6 by 3-inch cake pan and set aside.

2. In a small bowl, use a fork to whisk together the eggs, almond milk, salt, and pepper. Add the ham, bell peppers, and green onions. Pour the mixture into the greased pan. Add the cheese on top (if using).

3. Place the pan in the basket of the air fryer. Cook for 8 minutes, or until the eggs are cooked to your liking.

4. Loosen the omelet from the sides of the pan with a spatula and place it on a serving plate. Garnish with green onions and serve with cherry tomatoes, if desired. Best served fresh.

busy family tip: *I've always been a planner, so whenever I want an omelet for breakfast, I chop and prep my fillings the night before. In the morning, all I have to do is pop the pan in the air fryer! It's much faster and easier than using the stovetop, and my family agrees that omelets made in the air fryer are the best and softest they've ever had.*

(per serving)   calories **476** | fat **32g** | protein **41g** | total carbs **3g** | fiber **1g**

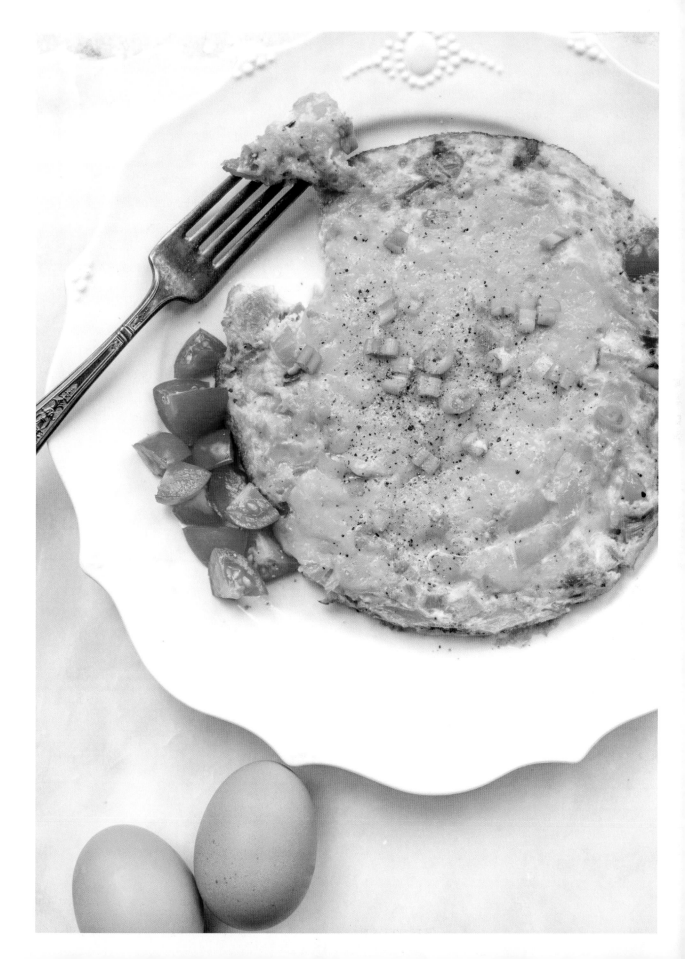

Easy Bacon

yield: 2 servings   *prep time:* 2 minutes   *cook time:* 6 minutes

4 slices thin-cut bacon or beef bacon

1. Spray the air fryer basket with avocado oil. Preheat the air fryer to 360°F.

2. Place the bacon in the air fryer basket in a single layer, spaced about ¼ inch apart. (I made mine into heart shapes and placed a small baking sheet on top to keep the shape.) Cook for 4 to 6 minutes (thicker bacon will take longer). Check the bacon after 4 minutes to make sure it is not overcooking.

3. Best served fresh. Store extras in an airtight container in the fridge for up to 4 days. Reheat in a preheated 360°F air fryer for 2 minutes, or until heated through.

(per serving)   calories **140** | fat **12g** | protein **8g** | total carbs **0g** | fiber **0g**

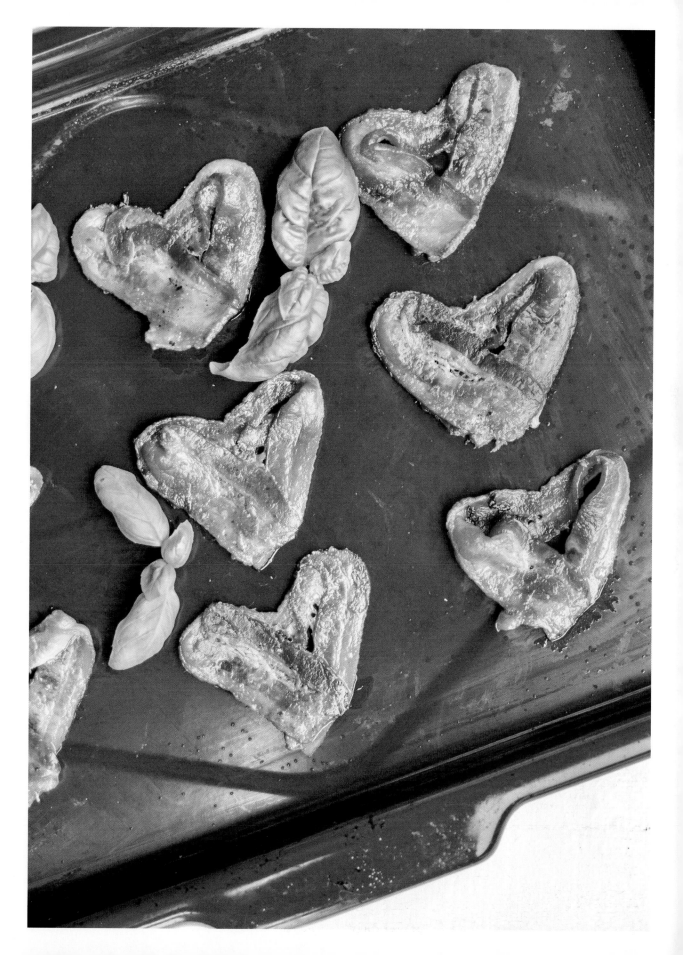

Valerie's Breakfast Sammies

yield: 5 servings   *prep time:* 15 minutes   *cook time:* 20 minutes

option   KETO

BISCUITS:

6 large egg whites

2 cups blanched almond flour, plus more if needed

1½ teaspoons baking powder

½ teaspoon fine sea salt

¼ cup (½ stick) very cold unsalted butter (or lard for dairy-free), cut into ¼-inch pieces (see Tip)

EGGS:

5 large eggs

½ teaspoon fine sea salt

¼ teaspoon ground black pepper

5 (1-ounce) slices cheddar cheese (omit for dairy-free)

10 thin slices ham, or 4 cooked Gyro Breakfast Patties (page 36)

1. Spray the air fryer basket with avocado oil. Preheat the air fryer to 350°F. Grease two 6-inch pie pans or two baking pans that will fit inside your air fryer.

2. Make the biscuits: In a medium-sized bowl, whip the egg whites with a hand mixer until very stiff. Set aside.

3. In a separate medium-sized bowl, stir together the almond flour, baking powder, and salt until well combined. Cut in the butter. Gently fold the flour mixture into the egg whites with a rubber spatula. If the dough is too wet to form into mounds, add a few tablespoons of almond flour until the dough holds together well.

4. Using a large spoon, divide the dough into 5 equal portions and drop them about 1 inch apart on one of the greased pie pans. (If you're using a smaller air fryer, work in batches if necessary.) Place the pan in the air fryer and cook for 11 to 14 minutes, until the biscuits are golden brown. Remove from the air fryer and set aside to cool.

5. Make the eggs: Set the air fryer to 375°F. Crack the eggs into the remaining greased pie pan and sprinkle with the salt and pepper. Place the eggs in the air fryer to cook for 5 minutes, or until they are cooked to your liking.

6. Open the air fryer and top each egg yolk with a slice of cheese (if using). Cook for another minute, or until the cheese is melted.

7. Once the biscuits are cool, slice them in half lengthwise. Place 1 cooked egg topped with cheese and 2 slices of ham in each biscuit.

8. Store leftover biscuits, eggs, and ham in separate airtight containers in the fridge for up to 3 days. Reheat the biscuits and eggs on a baking sheet in a preheated 350°F air fryer for 5 minutes, or until warmed through.

tip: Make sure that the butter for the biscuits is very cold; if it's not, the biscuits won't turn out.

note: This recipe is named for Valerie Bertinelli, who made my biscuits into breakfast sammies and gave me the idea for this air fryer recipe!

(per serving)   calories **269** | fat **19g** | protein **22g** | total carbs **1g** | fiber **0g**
(biscuits only) calories **316** | fat **27g** | protein **14g** | total carbs **10g** | fiber **5g**

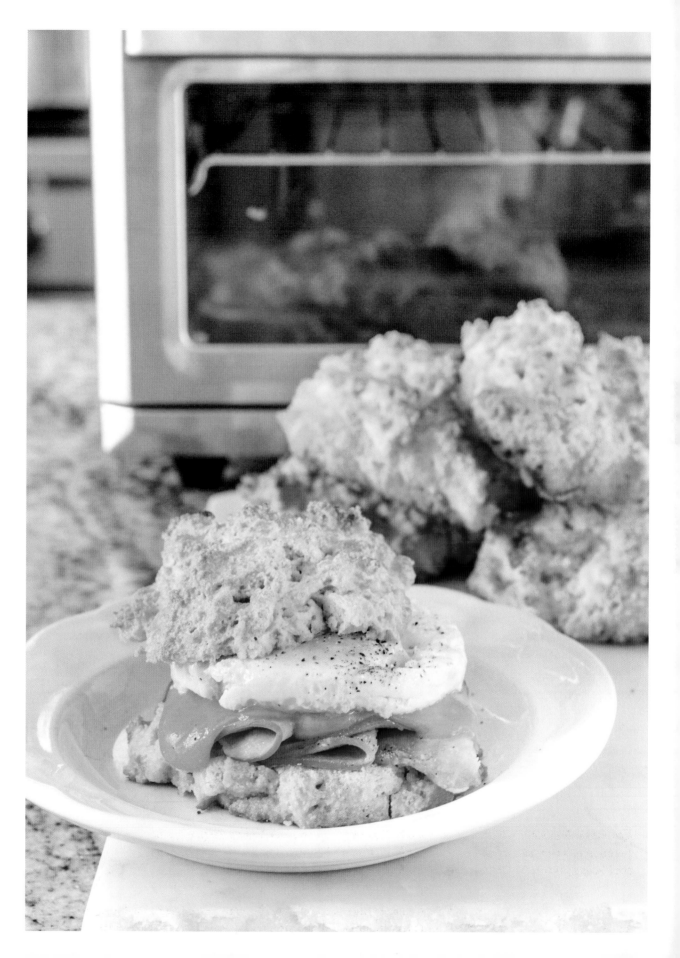

Gyro Breakfast Patties with Tzatziki

yield: 16 patties (2 per serving) *prep time:* 10 minutes *cook time:* 20 minutes per batch

PATTIES:

2 pounds ground lamb or beef

½ cup diced red onions

¼ cup sliced black olives

2 tablespoons tomato sauce

1 teaspoon dried oregano leaves

1 teaspoon Greek seasoning

2 cloves garlic, minced

1 teaspoon fine sea salt

TZATZIKI:

1 cup full-fat sour cream

1 small cucumber, chopped

½ teaspoon fine sea salt

½ teaspoon garlic powder,
or 1 clove garlic, minced

¼ teaspoon dried dill weed,
or 1 teaspoon finely chopped fresh
dill

FOR GARNISH/SERVING:

½ cup crumbled feta cheese
(about 2 ounces)

Diced red onions

Sliced black olives

Sliced cucumbers

1. Preheat the air fryer to 350°F.

2. Place the ground lamb, onions, olives, tomato sauce, oregano, Greek seasoning, garlic, and salt in a large bowl. Mix well to combine the ingredients.

3. Using your hands, form the mixture into sixteen 3-inch patties. Place about 5 of the patties in the air fryer and fry for 20 minutes, flipping halfway through. Remove the patties and place them on a serving platter. Repeat with the remaining patties.

4. While the patties cook, make the tzatziki: Place all the ingredients in a small bowl and stir well. Cover and store in the fridge until ready to serve. Garnish with ground black pepper before serving.

5. Serve the patties with a dollop of tzatziki, a sprinkle of crumbled feta cheese, diced red onions, sliced black olives, and sliced cucumbers.

6. Store leftovers in an airtight container in the refrigerator for up to 5 days or in the freezer for up to a month. Reheat the patties in a preheated 390°F air fryer for a few minutes, until warmed through.

busy family tip: *Make a double batch of this recipe and store the cooked patties in the fridge or freezer for easy breakfasts on the go.*

(per serving)   calories **396** | fat **31g** | protein **23g** | total carbs **4g** | fiber **0.4g**

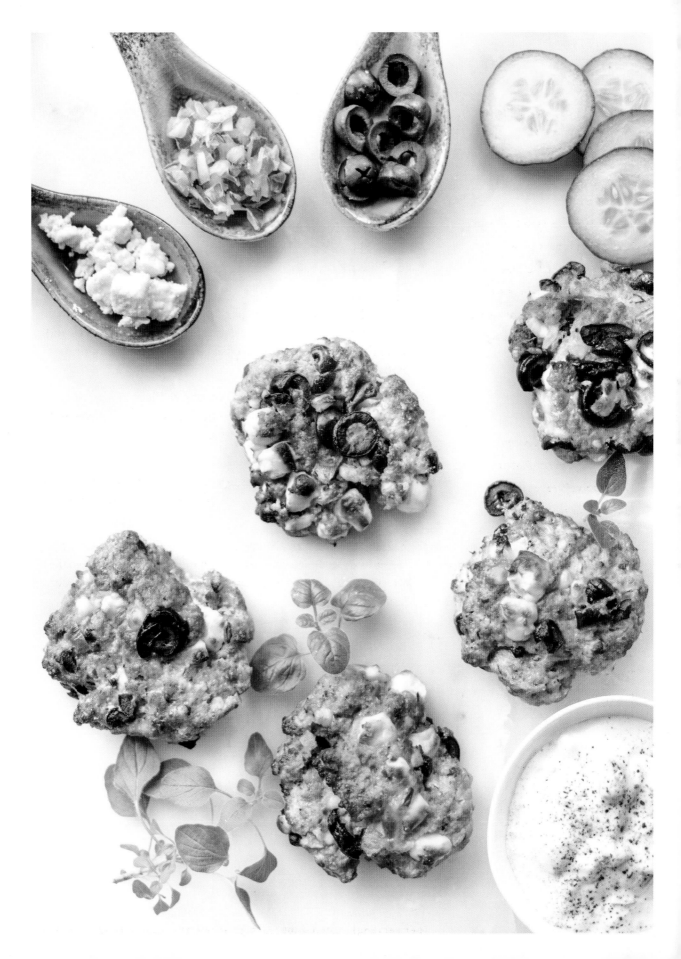

The Best Keto Quiche

yield: one 6-inch quiche (8 servings) *prep time:* 10 minutes *cook time:* 1 hour

CRUST:

1¼ cups blanched almond flour

1¼ cups grated Parmesan or Gouda cheese (about 3¾ ounces)

¼ teaspoon fine sea salt

1 large egg, beaten

FILLING:

½ cup chicken or beef broth (or vegetable broth for vegetarian)

1 cup shredded Swiss cheese (about 4 ounces)

4 ounces cream cheese (½ cup)

1 tablespoon unsalted butter, melted

4 large eggs, beaten

⅓ cup minced leeks or sliced green onions

¾ teaspoon fine sea salt

⅛ teaspoon cayenne pepper

Chopped green onions, for garnish

1. Preheat the air fryer to 325°F. Grease a 6-inch pie pan. Spray two large pieces of parchment paper with avocado oil and set them on the countertop.

2. Make the crust: In a medium-sized bowl, combine the flour, cheese, and salt and mix well. Add the egg and mix until the dough is well combined and stiff.

3. Place the dough in the center of one of the greased pieces of parchment. Top with the other piece of parchment. Using a rolling pin, roll out the dough into a circle about 1⁄16 inch thick.

4. Press the pie crust into the prepared pie pan. Place it in the air fryer and bake for 12 minutes, or until it starts to lightly brown.

5. While the crust bakes, make the filling: In a large bowl, combine the broth, Swiss cheese, cream cheese, and butter. Stir in the eggs, leeks, salt, and cayenne pepper. When the crust is ready, pour the mixture into the crust.

6. Place the quiche in the air fryer and bake for 15 minutes. Turn the heat down to 300°F and bake for an additional 30 minutes, or until a knife inserted 1 inch from the edge comes out clean. You may have to cover the edges of the crust with foil to prevent burning.

7. Allow the quiche to cool for 10 minutes before garnishing it with chopped green onions and cutting it into wedges.

8. Store leftovers in an airtight container in the refrigerator for up to 4 days or in the freezer for up to a month. Reheat in a preheated 350°F air fryer for a few minutes, until warmed through.

(per serving) calories **333** | fat **26g** | protein **20g** | total carbs **6g** | fiber **2g**

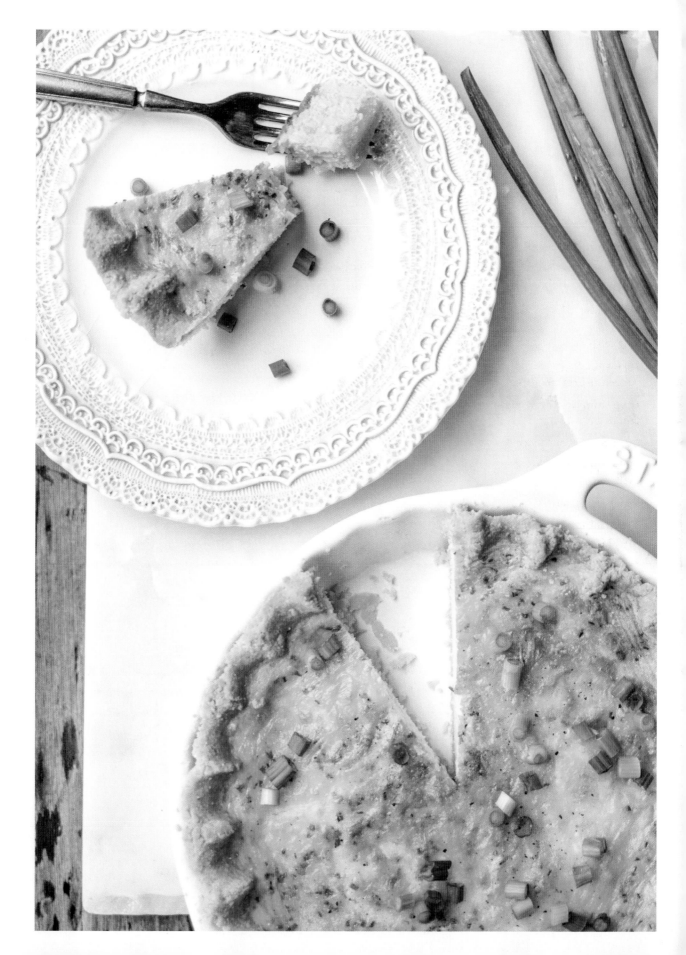

Easy Mexican Shakshuka

yield: 1 serving *prep time:* 5 minutes *cook time:* 6 minutes

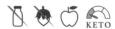

½ cup salsa

2 large eggs, room temperature

½ teaspoon fine sea salt

¼ teaspoon smoked paprika

⅛ teaspoon ground cumin

FOR GARNISH:

2 tablespoons cilantro leaves

1. Preheat the air fryer to 400°F.

2. Place the salsa in a 6-inch pie pan or a casserole dish that will fit into your air fryer. Crack the eggs into the salsa and sprinkle them with the salt, paprika, and cumin.

3. Place the pan in the air fryer and cook for 6 minutes, or until the egg whites are set and the yolks are cooked to your liking.

4. Remove from the air fryer and garnish with the cilantro before serving.

5. Best served fresh.

(per serving) calories **258** | fat **17g** | protein **14g** | total carbs **11g** | fiber **4g**

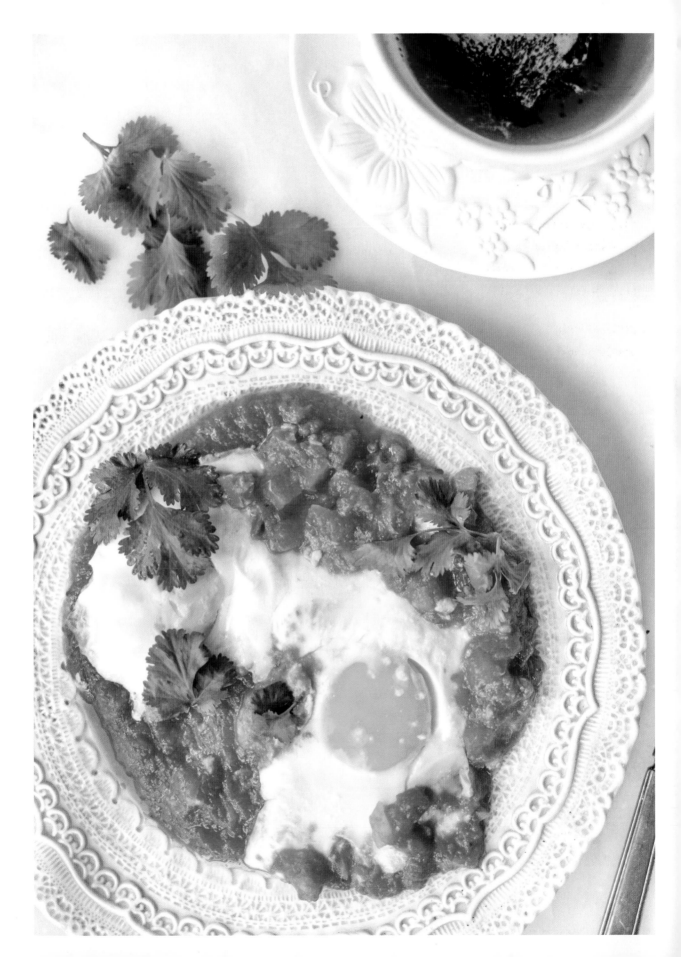

Green Eggs and Ham

yield: 2 servings   *prep time:* 5 minutes   *cook time:* 10 minutes

1 large Hass avocado, halved and pitted

2 thin slices ham

2 large eggs

2 tablespoons chopped green onions, plus more for garnish

½ teaspoon fine sea salt

¼ teaspoon ground black pepper

¼ cup shredded cheddar cheese (omit for dairy-free)

1. Preheat the air fryer to 400°F.

2. Place a slice of ham into the cavity of each avocado half. Crack an egg on top of the ham, then sprinkle on the green onions, salt, and pepper.

3. Place the avocado halves in the air fryer cut side up and cook for 10 minutes, or until the egg is cooked to your desired doneness. Top with the cheese (if using) and cook for 30 seconds more, or until the cheese is melted. Garnish with chopped green onions.

4. Best served fresh. Store extras in an airtight container in the fridge for up to 4 days. Reheat in a preheated 350°F air fryer for a few minutes, until warmed through.

(per serving)   calories **307** | fat **24g** | protein **14g** | total carbs **10g** | fiber **7g**

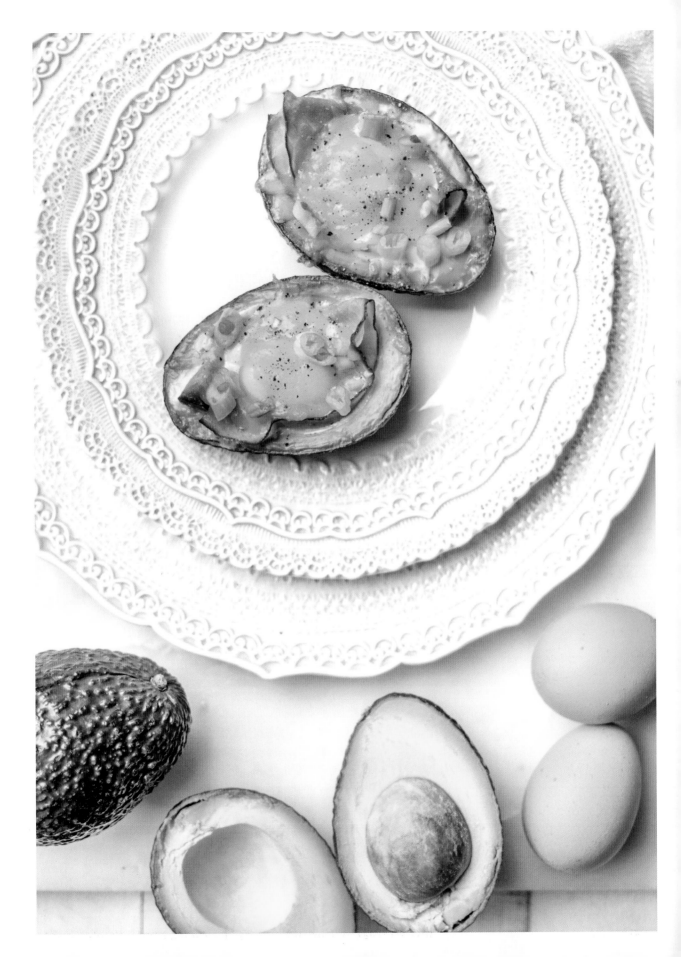

Everything Bagels

yield: 6 bagels (1 per serving)   *prep time:* 15 minutes   *cook time:* 14 minutes

KETO

1¾ cups shredded mozzarella cheese or goat cheese mozzarella

2 tablespoons unsalted butter or coconut oil

1 large egg, beaten

1 tablespoon apple cider vinegar

1 cup blanched almond flour

1 tablespoon baking powder

⅛ teaspoon fine sea salt

1½ teaspoons everything bagel seasoning

1. Make the dough: Put the mozzarella and butter in a large microwave-safe bowl and microwave for 1 to 2 minutes, until the cheese is entirely melted. Stir well. Add the egg and vinegar. Using a hand mixer on medium, combine well. Add the almond flour, baking powder, and salt and, using the mixer, combine well.

2. Lay a piece of parchment paper on the countertop and place the dough on it. Knead it for about 3 minutes. The dough should be a little sticky but pliable. (If the dough is too sticky, chill it in the refrigerator for an hour or overnight.)

3. Preheat the air fryer to 350°F. Spray a baking sheet or pie pan that will fit into your air fryer with avocado oil.

4. Divide the dough into 6 equal portions. Roll 1 portion into a log that is 6 inches long and about ½ inch thick. Form the log into a circle and seal the edges together, making a bagel shape. Repeat with the remaining portions of dough, making 6 bagels.

5. Place the bagels on the greased baking sheet. Spray the bagels with avocado oil and top with everything bagel seasoning, pressing the seasoning into the dough with your hands.

6. Place the bagels in the air fryer and cook for 14 minutes, or until cooked through and golden brown, flipping after 6 minutes.

7. Remove the bagels from the air fryer and allow them to cool slightly before slicing them in half and serving. Store leftovers in an airtight container in the fridge for up to 4 days or in the freezer for up to a month.

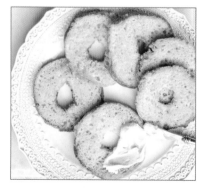

tips: This dough is very forgiving. If it cracks while you're forming the bagels, use your hands to press any cracks together. The bagels will puff up, so when you're forming them, make sure the circle in the middle is large—otherwise it may close up during baking.

Bagel chips are a great snack, and they're easy to make with these bagels. Slice a bagel into ¼-inch-thick rounds and spread each round with 1 teaspoon unsalted butter. Place the rounds in the air fryer in a single layer, leaving space between them, and cook for 5 to 6 minutes, until crispy. They're best served fresh, but they'll keep in an airtight container in the fridge for up to 4 days or in the freezer for up to a month.

(per serving)   calories **224** | fat **19g** | protein **12g** | total carbs **4g** | fiber **2g**

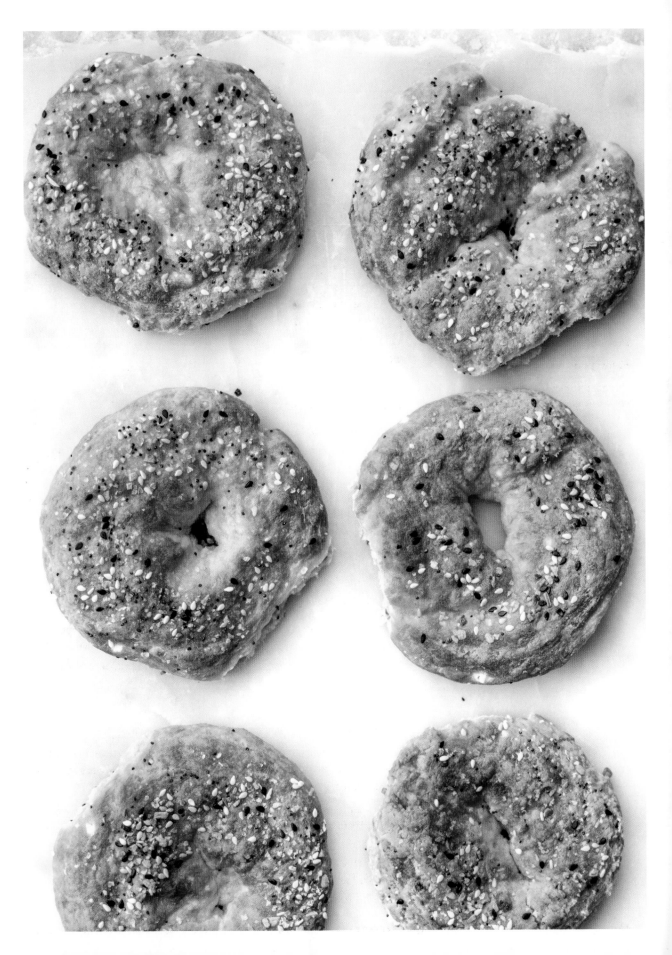

Keto Danish

yield: 6 Danish (1 per serving)   *prep time:* 15 minutes   *cook time:* 20 minutes

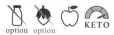

PASTRY:

3 large eggs

¼ teaspoon cream of tartar

¼ cup vanilla-flavored egg white protein powder

¼ cup Swerve confectioners'-style sweetener or equivalent amount of liquid or powdered sweetener (see page 18), or 1 teaspoon stevia glycerite

3 tablespoons full-fat sour cream (or coconut cream for dairy-free)

1 teaspoon vanilla extract

FILLING:

4 ounces cream cheese (½ cup) (or Kite Hill brand cream cheese style spread for dairy-free), softened

2 large egg yolks (from above)

¼ cup Swerve confectioners'-style sweetener or equivalent amount of liquid or powdered sweetener (see page 18), or ½ teaspoon stevia glycerite

1 teaspoon vanilla extract

¼ teaspoon ground cinnamon

DRIZZLE:

1 ounce cream cheese (2 tablespoons) (or Kite Hill brand cream cheese style spread for dairy-free), softened

1 tablespoon Swerve confectioners'-style sweetener or equivalent amount of liquid or powdered sweetener (see page 18), or 1 drop stevia glycerite

1 tablespoon unsweetened, unflavored almond milk (or heavy cream for nut-free)

1. Preheat the air fryer to 300°F. Spray a casserole dish that will fit in your air fryer with avocado oil.

2. Make the pastry: Separate the eggs, putting all the whites in a large bowl, one yolk in a medium-sized bowl, and two yolks in a small bowl. Beat all the egg yolks and set aside.

3. Add the cream of tartar to the egg whites. Whip the whites with a hand mixer until very stiff, then turn the hand mixer's setting to low and slowly add the protein powder while mixing. Mix until only just combined; if you mix too long, the whites will fall. Set aside.

4. To the egg yolk in the medium-sized bowl, add the sweetener, sour cream, and vanilla extract. Mix well. Slowly pour the yolk mixture into the egg whites and gently combine. Dollop 6 equal-sized mounds of batter into the casserole dish. Use the back of a large spoon to make an indentation on the top of each mound. Set aside.

5. Make the filling: Place the cream cheese in a small bowl and stir to break it up. Add the 2 remaining egg yolks, the sweetener, vanilla extract, and cinnamon and stir until well combined. Divide the filling among the mounds of batter, pouring it into the indentations on the tops.

6. Place the Danish in the air fryer and bake for about 20 minutes, or until golden brown.

7. While the Danish bake, make the drizzle: In a small bowl, stir the cream cheese to break it up. Stir in the sweetener and almond milk. Place the mixture in a piping bag or a small resealable plastic bag with one corner snipped off. After the Danish have cooled, pipe the drizzle over the Danish.

8. Store leftovers in airtight container in the fridge for up to 4 days.

(per serving)   calories **160** | fat **12g** | protein **8g** | total carbs **2g** | fiber **0.3g**

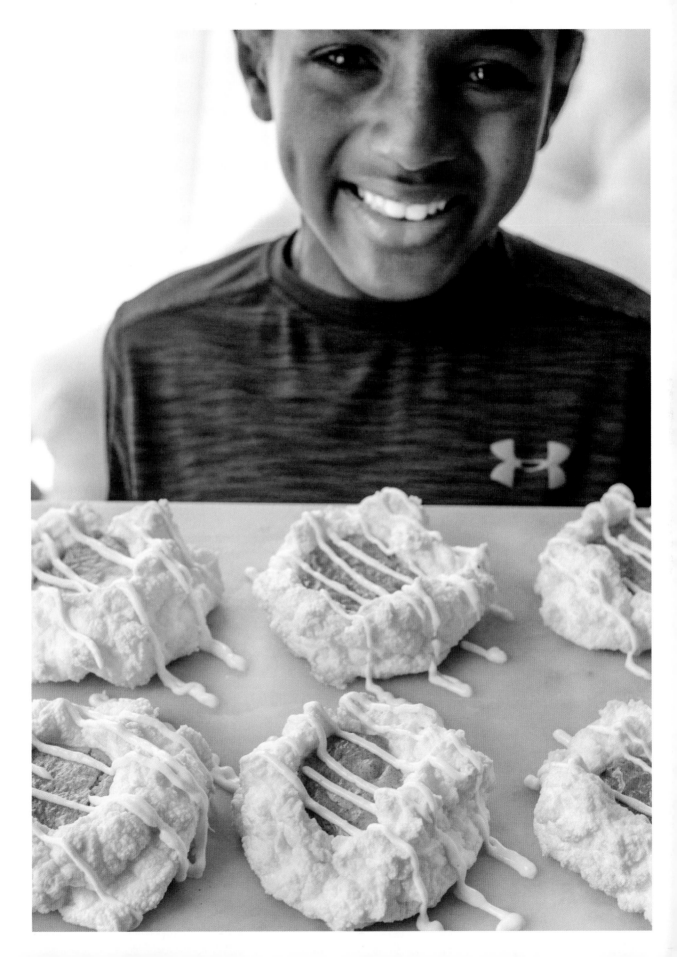

French Toast Pavlova

yield: one 7-inch cake (4 servings)
prep time: 15 minutes, plus 20 minutes to rest and 20 minutes to chill *cook time:* 1 hour

3 large egg whites

¼ teaspoon cream of tartar

¾ cup Swerve confectioners'-style sweetener or equivalent amount of powdered sweetener (see page 18)

1 teaspoon ground cinnamon

1 teaspoon maple extract

TOPPINGS:

½ cup heavy cream

3 tablespoons Swerve confectioners'-style sweetener or equivalent amount of powdered sweetener (see page 18), plus more for garnish

Fresh strawberries (optional)

note: Meringues and humidity do not mix. If your kitchen is very humid, the outside of the meringue won't crisp up.

1. Preheat the air fryer to 275°F. Thoroughly grease a 7-inch pie pan with butter or coconut oil. Place a large bowl in the refrigerator to chill.

2. In a small bowl, combine the egg whites and cream of tartar. Using a hand mixer, beat until soft peaks form. Turn the mixer to low and slowly sprinkle in the sweetener while mixing until completely incorporated. Add the cinnamon and maple extract and beat on medium-high until the peaks become stiff.

3. Spoon the mixture into the greased pie pan, then smooth it across the bottom, up the sides, and onto the rim of the pie pan to form a shell. Cook in the air fryer for 1 hour, then turn off the air fryer and let the shell stand in the air fryer for another 20 minutes. Once the shell has set, transfer it to the refrigerator to chill for 20 minutes or the freezer to chill for 10 minutes.

4. While the shell sets and chills, make the topping: Remove the large bowl from the refrigerator and place the heavy cream in it. Whip with a hand mixer on high until soft peaks form. Add the sweetener and beat until medium peaks form. Taste and adjust the sweetness to your liking.

5. Place the chilled shell on a serving platter and spoon on the cream topping. Top with the strawberries, if desired, and garnish with powdered sweetener. Slice and serve.

6. If you won't be eating the pavlova right away, store the shell and topping in separate airtight containers in the refrigerator for up to 3 days.

(per serving) calories **115** | fat **11g** | protein **3g** | total carbs **2g** | fiber **0.3g**

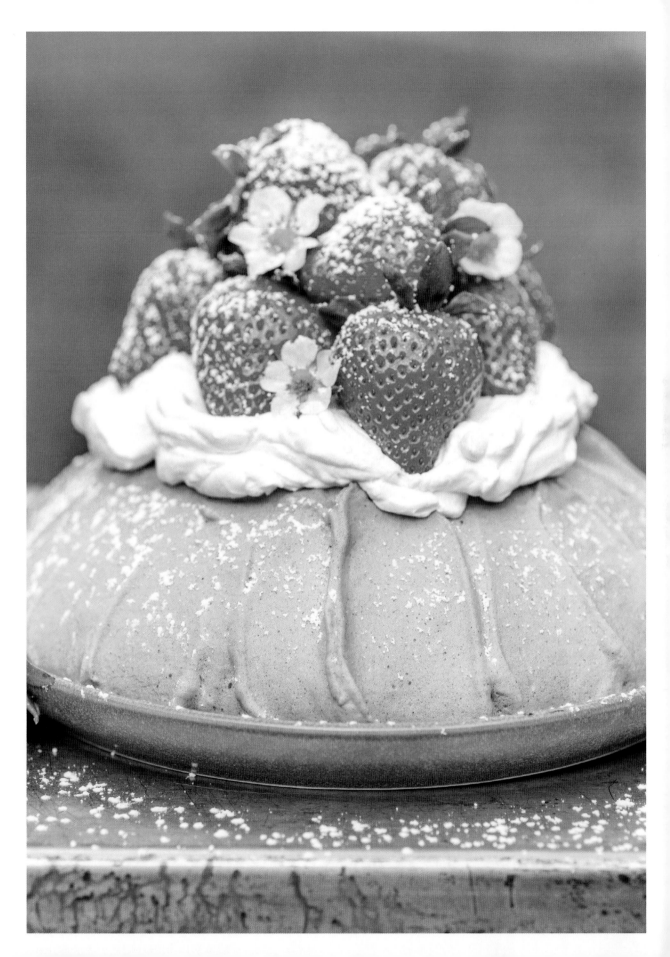

Breakfast Cobbler

yield: 4 servings   *prep time:* 20 minutes   *cook time:* 30 minutes

KETO

FILLING:

10 ounces bulk pork sausage, crumbled

¼ cup minced onions

2 cloves garlic, minced

½ teaspoon fine sea salt

½ teaspoon ground black pepper

1 (8-ounce) package cream cheese (or Kite Hill brand cream cheese style spread for dairy-free), softened

¾ cup beef or chicken broth

BISCUITS:

3 large egg whites

¾ cup blanched almond flour

1 teaspoon baking powder

¼ teaspoon fine sea salt

2½ tablespoons very cold unsalted butter, cut into ¼-inch pieces (see Tip)

Fresh thyme leaves, for garnish

tip: Make sure that the butter for the biscuits is very cold; if it's not, the biscuits won't turn out.

1. Preheat the air fryer to 400°F.

2. Place the sausage, onions, and garlic in a 7-inch pie pan. Using your hands, break up the sausage into small pieces and spread it evenly throughout the pie pan. Season with the salt and pepper. Place the pan in the air fryer and cook for 5 minutes.

3. While the sausage cooks, place the cream cheese and broth in a food processor or blender and puree until smooth.

4. Remove the pork from the air fryer and use a fork or metal spatula to crumble it more. Pour the cream cheese mixture into the sausage and stir to combine. Set aside.

5. Make the biscuits: Place the egg whites in a medium-sized mixing bowl or the bowl of a stand mixer and whip with a hand mixer or stand mixer until stiff peaks form.

6. In a separate medium-sized bowl, whisk together the almond flour, baking powder, and salt, then cut in the butter. When you are done, the mixture should still have chunks of butter. Gently fold the flour mixture into the egg whites with a rubber spatula.

7. Use a large spoon or ice cream scoop to scoop the dough into 4 equal-sized biscuits, making sure the butter is evenly distributed. Place the biscuits on top of the sausage and cook in the air fryer for 5 minutes, then turn the heat down to 325°F and cook for another 17 to 20 minutes, until the biscuits are golden brown. Serve garnished with fresh thyme leaves.

8. Store leftovers in an airtight container in the refrigerator for up to 3 days. Reheat in a preheated 350°F air fryer for 5 minutes, or until warmed through.

(per serving)   calories **623** | fat **55g** | protein **23g** | total carbs **8g** | fiber **3g**

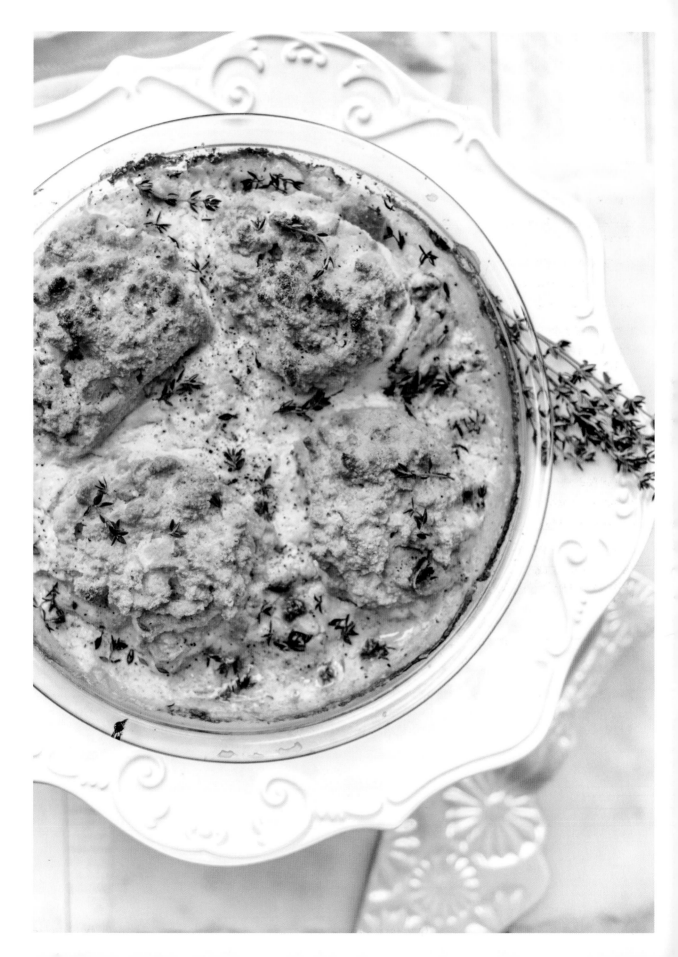

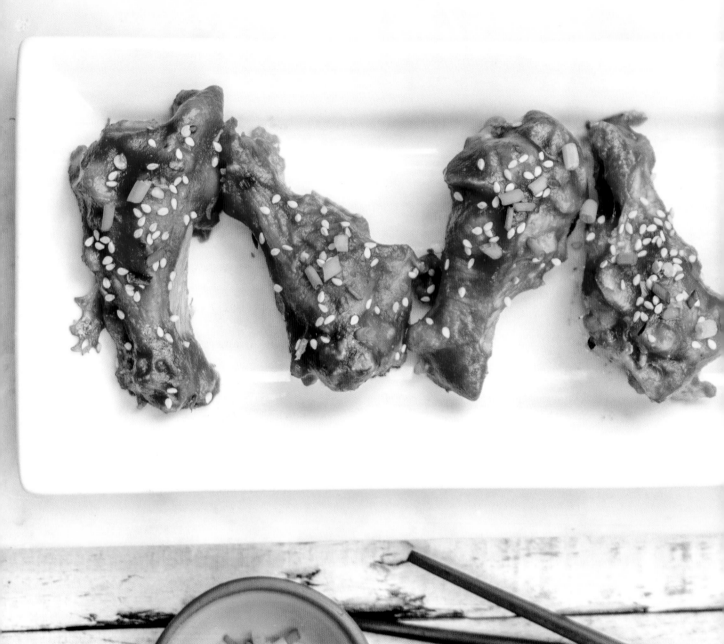
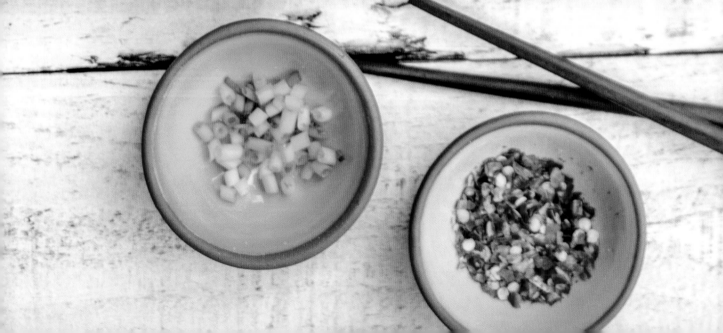

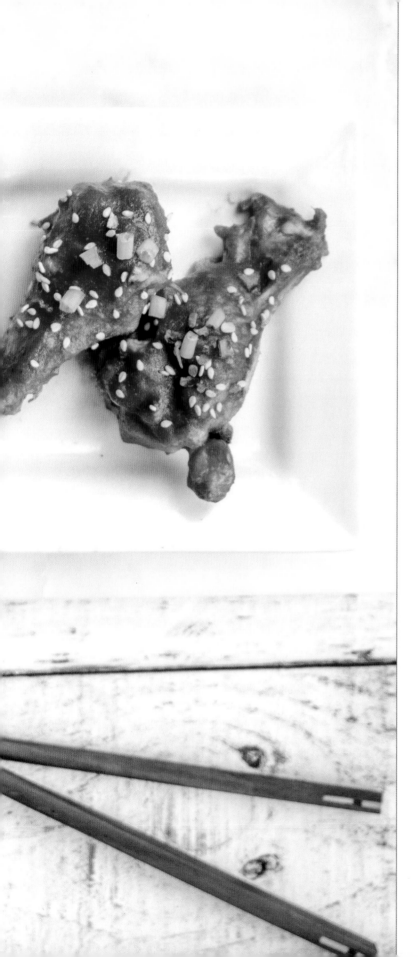

Appetizers

Buffalo Cauliflower

yield: 4 servings   *prep time:* 5 minutes   *cook time:* 11 minutes

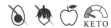

¼ cup hot sauce

¼ cup powdered Parmesan cheese (see page 19)

2 tablespoons unsalted butter, melted

1 small head cauliflower, cut into 1-inch bites

Blue Cheese Dressing (see below), for serving

1. Preheat the air fryer to 400°F. Spray a baking dish that will fit into your air fryer with avocado oil.

2. Place the hot sauce, Parmesan, and butter in a large bowl and stir to combine. Add the cauliflower and toss to coat well.

3. Place the coated cauliflower in the baking dish. Cook in the air fryer for 11 minutes, stirring halfway through. Serve with blue cheese dressing.

4. Store leftovers in an airtight container in the fridge for up to 4 days. Reheat in a preheated 400°F oven for 3 minutes, until warmed through and crispy.

Blue Cheese Dressing

makes: about 2 cups (2 tablespoons per serving)

8 ounces crumbled blue cheese, plus more if desired for a chunky texture

¼ cup beef bone broth

¼ cup full-fat sour cream

¼ cup red wine vinegar or coconut vinegar

1½ tablespoons Swerve confectioners'-style sweetener or equivalent amount of liquid or powdered sweetener (see page 18)

1 tablespoon MCT oil

1 clove garlic, peeled

Place all the ingredients in a food processor and blend until smooth. Transfer to a jar. Stir in extra chunks of blue cheese if desired. Store in the refrigerator for up to 5 days.

(per serving)   calories **185** | fat **15g** | protein **9g** | total carbs **4g** | fiber **2g**

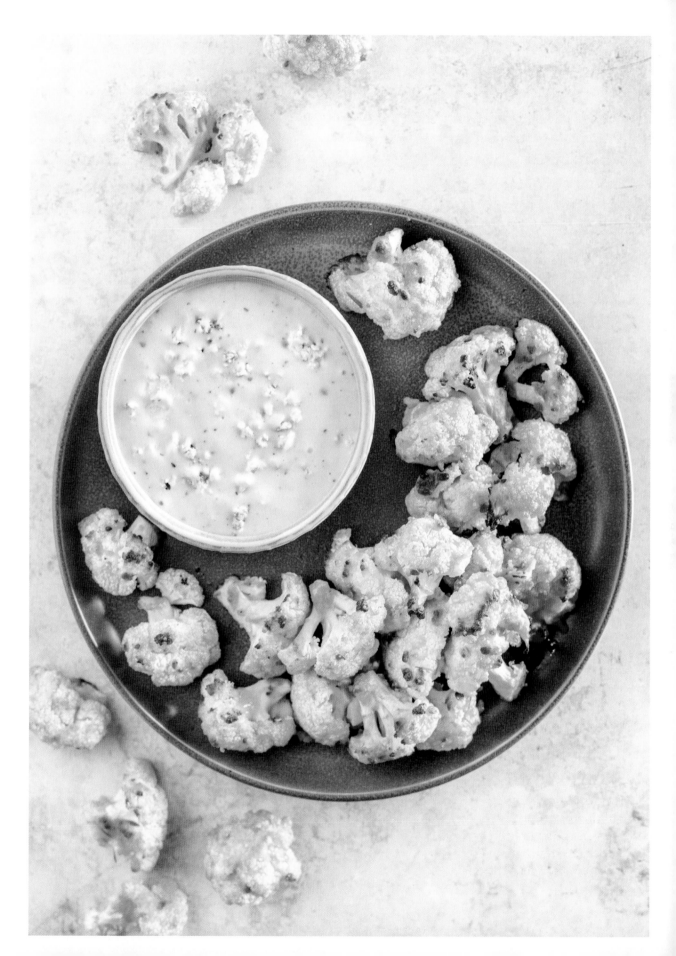

Ranch Kale Chips

yield: 8 cups (½ cup per serving) *prep time:* 5 minutes *cook time:* 10 minutes per batch

½ teaspoon dried chives

½ teaspoon dried dill weed

½ teaspoon dried parsley

¼ teaspoon garlic powder

¼ teaspoon onion powder

⅛ teaspoon fine sea salt

⅛ teaspoon ground black pepper

2 large bunches kale

1. Spray the air fryer basket with avocado oil. Preheat the air fryer to 360°F.

2. Place the seasonings, salt, and pepper in a small bowl and mix well.

3. Wash the kale and pat completely dry. Use a sharp knife to carve out the thick inner stems, then spray the leaves with avocado oil and sprinkle them with the seasoning mix.

4. Place the kale leaves in the air fryer in a single layer and cook for 10 minutes, shaking and rotating the chips halfway through. Transfer the baked chips to a baking sheet to cool completely and crisp up. Repeat with the remaining kale. Sprinkle the cooled chips with salt before serving, if desired.

5. Kale chips can be stored in an airtight container at room temperature for up to 1 week, but they are best eaten within 3 days.

(per serving) calories **11** | fat **0.2g** | protein **1g** | total carbs **2g** | fiber **0.4g**

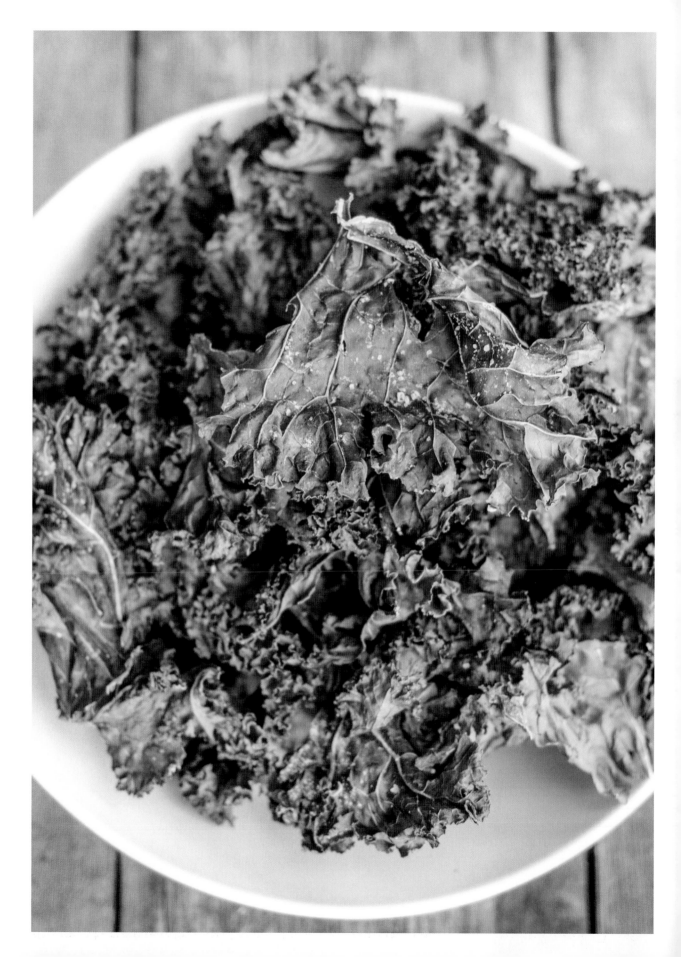

Crispy Nacho Avocado Fries

yield: 6 servings *prep time:* 10 minutes *cook time:* 15 minutes

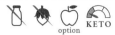

3 firm, barely ripe avocados, halved, peeled, and pitted (see Tip)

2 cups pork dust (see page 19) (or powdered Parmesan cheese for vegetarian; see page 19)

2 teaspoons fine sea salt

2 teaspoons ground black pepper

2 teaspoons ground cumin

1 teaspoon chili powder

1 teaspoon paprika

½ teaspoon garlic powder

½ teaspoon onion powder

2 large eggs

Salsa, for serving (optional)

Fresh chopped cilantro leaves, for garnish (optional)

1. Spray the air fryer basket with avocado oil. Preheat the air fryer to 400°F.

2. Slice the avocados into thick-cut french fry shapes.

3. In a bowl, mix together the pork dust, salt, pepper, and seasonings.

4. In a separate shallow bowl, beat the eggs.

5. Dip the avocado fries into the beaten eggs and shake off any excess, then dip them into the pork dust mixture. Use your hands to press the breading into each fry.

6. Spray the fries with avocado oil and place them in the air fryer basket in a single layer, leaving space between them. If there are too many fries to fit in a single layer, work in batches. Cook in the air fryer for 13 to 15 minutes, until golden brown, flipping after 5 minutes.

7. Serve with salsa, if desired, and garnish with fresh chopped cilantro, if desired. Best served fresh.

8. Store leftovers in an airtight container in the fridge for up to 5 days. Reheat in a preheated 400°F air fryer for 3 minutes, or until heated through.

tip: Avocados may seem like an odd replacement for potatoes, but baked avocado fries truly have a french fry–like texture. When purchasing avocados for this recipe, choose firm ones so they are easy to slice.

(per serving) calories **282** | fat **22g** | protein **15g** | total carbs **9g** | fiber **7g**

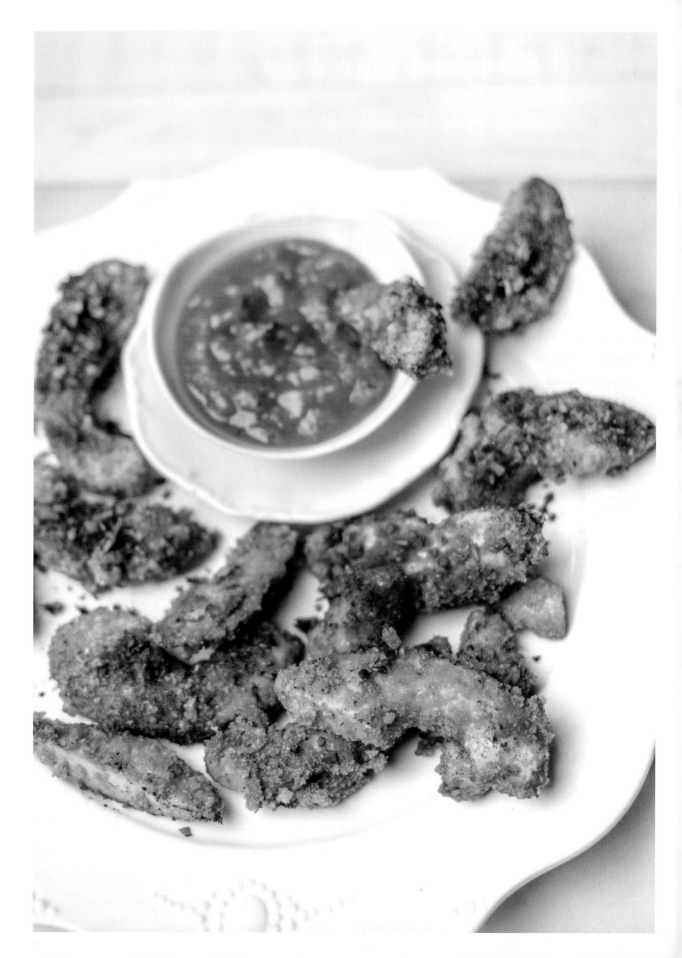

Bacon-Wrapped Pickle Poppers

yield: 24 poppers (4 per serving)   *prep time:* 10 minutes   *cook time:* 10 minutes

12 medium dill pickles

1 (8-ounce) package cream cheese, softened

1 cup shredded sharp cheddar cheese (about 4 ounces)

12 slices bacon or beef bacon, sliced in half lengthwise

Ranch Dressing (page 68) or Blue Cheese Dressing (page 54), for serving (optional)

1. Spray the air fryer basket with avocado oil. Preheat the air fryer to 400°F.

2. Slice the dill pickles in half lengthwise and use a spoon to scoop out the centers.

3. Place the cream cheese and cheddar cheese in a small bowl and stir until well combined.

4. Divide the cream cheese mixture among the pickles, spooning equal amounts into the scooped-out centers. Wrap each filled pickle with a slice of bacon and secure the bacon with toothpicks.

5. Place the bacon-wrapped pickles in the air fryer basket with the bacon seam side down and cook for 8 to 10 minutes, until the bacon is crispy, flipping halfway through. Serve warm with ranch or blue cheese dressing, if desired.

6. Best served fresh. Store leftovers in an airtight container in the fridge for up to 5 days. Reheat in a preheated 400°F air fryer for 3 minutes, or until heated through.

tip: One of my recipe testers skipped the step of securing bacon with toothpicks, and the filling fell out when she flipped the poppers. Do not skip that step.

(per serving)   calories **87** | fat **8g** | protein **4g** | total carbs **1g** | fiber **?g**

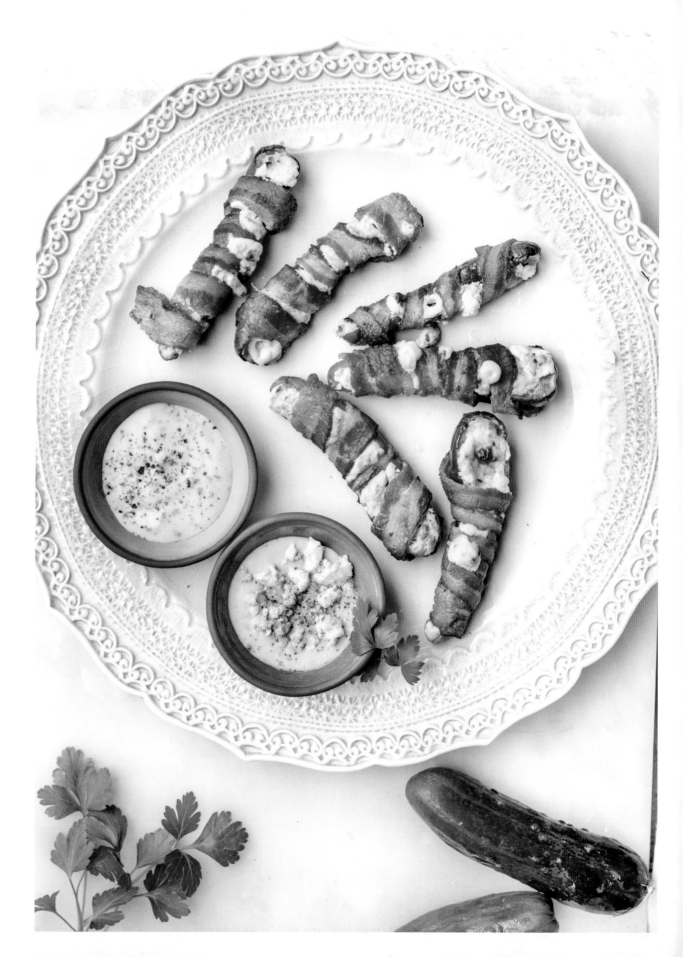

Bourbon Chicken Wings

yield: 8 servings *prep time:* 10 minutes *cook time:* 32 minutes

2 pounds chicken wings or drummies

½ teaspoon fine sea salt

SAUCE:

½ cup chicken broth

⅓ cup Swerve confectioners'-style sweetener or equivalent amount of liquid or powdered sweetener (see page 18)

¼ cup tomato sauce

¼ cup wheat-free tamari

1 tablespoon apple cider vinegar

¾ teaspoon red pepper flakes

¼ teaspoon grated fresh ginger

1 clove garlic, smashed to a paste

FOR GARNISH (OPTIONAL):

Chopped green onions

Sesame seeds

1. Spray the air fryer basket with avocado oil. Preheat the air fryer to 380°F.

2. Season the chicken wings on all sides with the salt and place them in the air fryer. Cook for 25 minutes, flipping after 15 minutes. After 25 minutes, increase the temperature to 400°F and cook for 6 to 7 minutes more, until the skin is browned and crisp.

3. While the wings cook, make the sauce: Place all the sauce ingredients in a large sauté pan and whisk to combine. Simmer until reduced and thickened, about 10 minutes.

4. Brush the cooked chicken wings with the sauce. Garnish with green onions and sesame seeds, if desired. Serve with extra sauce on the side for dipping.

5. Store leftovers in an airtight container in the refrigerator for up to 4 days. Reheat in a preheated 350°F air fryer for 5 minutes, then increase the temperature to 400°F and cook for 3 to 5 more minutes, until warm and crispy.

(per serving) calories **545** | fat **30g** | protein **42g** | total carbs **3g** | fiber **0.1g**

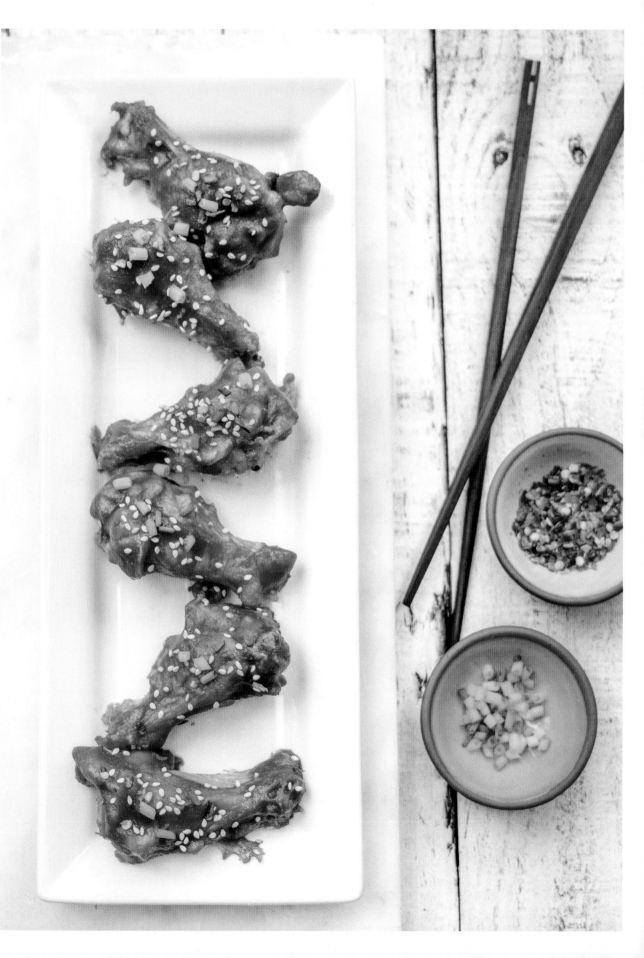

Doro Wat Wings

yield: 1 dozen wings (6 per serving)   *prep time:* 5 minutes   *cook time:* 32 minutes

1 dozen chicken wings or drummies

1 tablespoon coconut oil or bacon fat, melted

2 teaspoons berbere spice

1 teaspoon fine sea salt

FOR SERVING
(OMIT FOR EGG-FREE):

2 hard-boiled eggs

½ teaspoon fine sea salt

¼ teaspoon berbere spice

¼ teaspoon dried chives

1. Spray the air fryer basket with avocado oil. Preheat the air fryer to 380°F.

2. Place the chicken wings in a large bowl. Pour the oil over them and turn to coat completely. Sprinkle the berbere and salt on all sides of the chicken.

3. Place the chicken wings in the air fryer and cook for 25 minutes, flipping after 15 minutes.

4. After 25 minutes, increase the temperature to 400°F and cook for 6 to 7 minutes more, until the skin is browned and crisp.

5. While the chicken cooks, prepare the hard-boiled eggs (if using): Peel the eggs, slice them in half, and season them with the salt, berbere, and dried chives. Serve the chicken and eggs together.

6. Store leftovers in an airtight container in the fridge for up to 4 days. Reheat the chicken in a preheated 400°F air fryer for 5 minutes, or until heated through.

(per serving)   calories **317** | fat **24g** | protein **24g** | total carbs **0.1g** | fiber **0g**

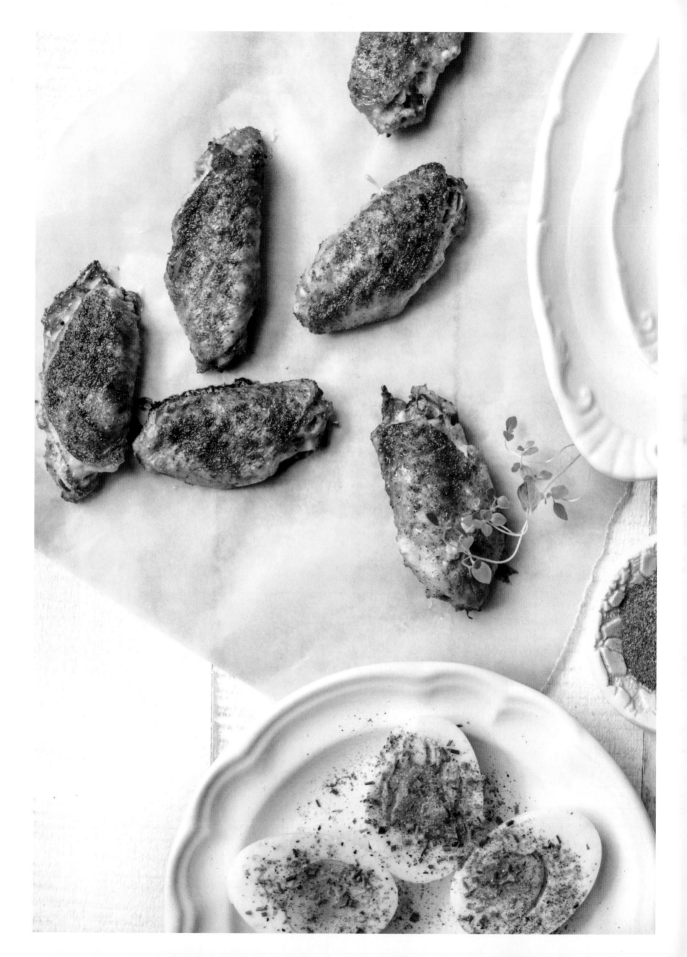

Salt and Vinegar Pork Belly Chips

yield: 4 servings   *prep time:* 5 minutes, plus 30 minutes to marinate   *cook time:* 12 minutes

1 pound slab pork belly (see Tip)

½ cup apple cider vinegar

Fine sea salt

FOR SERVING (OPTIONAL):

Guacamole

Pico de gallo

busy family tip: You can get fully cooked pork belly from Trader Joe's; you need just one package for this recipe.

1. Slice the pork belly into ⅛-inch-thick strips and place them in a shallow dish. Pour in the vinegar and stir to coat the pork belly. Place in the fridge to marinate for 30 minutes.

2. Spray the air fryer basket with avocado oil. Preheat the air fryer to 400°F.

3. Remove the pork belly from the vinegar and place the strips in the air fryer basket in a single layer, leaving space between them. Cook in the air fryer for 10 to 12 minutes, until crispy, flipping after 5 minutes. Remove from the air fryer and sprinkle with salt. Serve with guacamole and pico de gallo, if desired.

4. Best served fresh. Store leftovers in an airtight container in the fridge for up to 5 days. Reheat in a preheated 400°F air fryer for 5 minutes, or until heated through, flipping halfway through.

(per serving)   calories **240** | fat **21g** | protein **13g** | total carbs **0g** | fiber **0g**

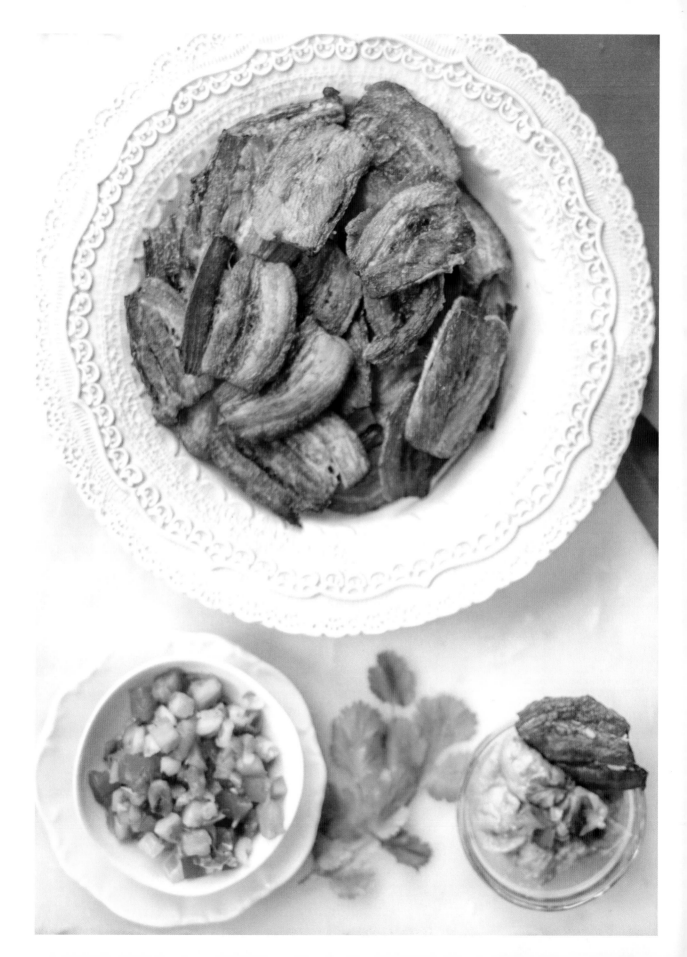

Crispy Prosciutto-Wrapped Onion Rings

yield: 6 servings   *prep time:* 10 minutes   *cook time:* 10 minutes

3 large sweet onions

24 slices prosciutto or beef bacon

1 cup Ranch Dressing (see below), for serving (optional; use dairy-free if needed)

1. Spray the air fryer basket with avocado oil. Preheat the air fryer to 400°F.

2. Cut the onions into ⅔-inch-thick slices. Reserve the small inside rings for other recipes; you want the large rings, which are easy to wrap in prosciutto.

3. Wrap each onion ring tightly in prosciutto. Place the wrapped onion rings into the air fryer and cook for 10 minutes, or until the prosciutto is crispy. Serve with ranch dressing, if desired.

4. Store leftovers in an airtight container in the fridge for up to 5 days. Reheat in a preheated 400°F air fryer for 5 minutes, or until heated through, flipping halfway through.

Ranch Dressing

makes: about 1½ cups

1 (8-ounce) package cream cheese (or Kite Hill brand cream cheese style spread for dairy-free), softened

½ cup chicken or beef broth

½ teaspoon dried chives

½ teaspoon dried dill weed

½ teaspoon dried parsley

¼ teaspoon garlic powder

¼ teaspoon onion powder

⅛ teaspoon fine sea salt

⅛ teaspoon ground black pepper

In a blender or using a hand mixer with a large bowl, mix together all the ingredients until well combined. Cover and refrigerate for 2 hours before serving (it will thicken up as it rests).

(per serving)   calories **318** | fat **28g** | protein **14g** | total carbs **3g** | fiber **0.4g**

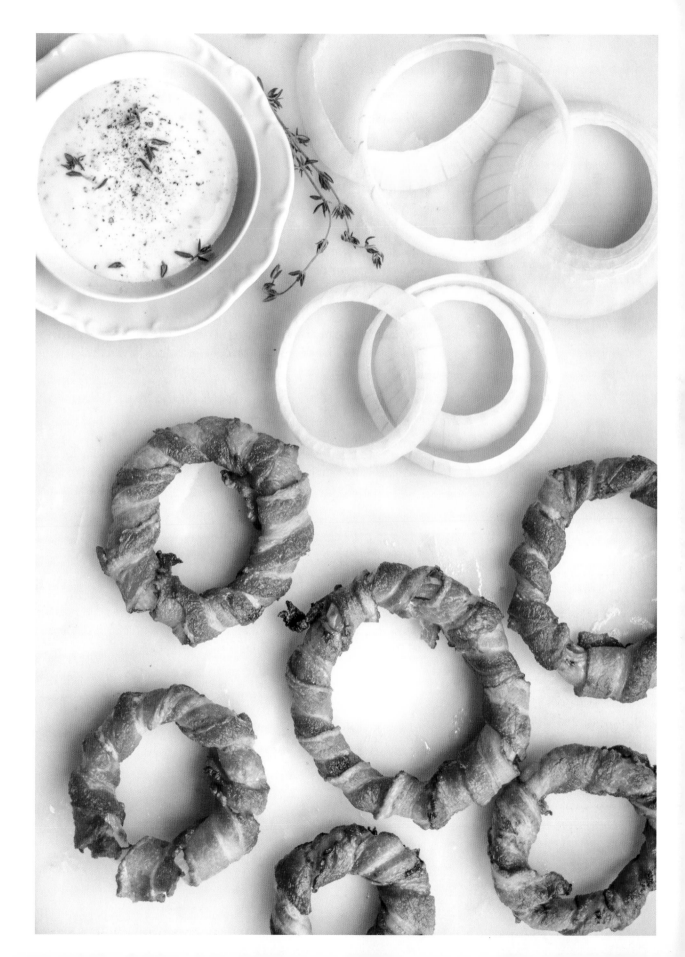

Bacon-Wrapped Asparagus

yield: 4 servings   *prep time:* 5 minutes   *cook time:* 10 minutes

1 pound asparagus, trimmed (about 24 spears)

4 slices bacon or beef bacon

½ cup Ranch Dressing (page 68), for serving

2 tablespoons chopped fresh chives, for garnish

1. Spray the air fryer basket with avocado oil. Preheat the air fryer to 400°F.

2. Slice the bacon down the middle, making long, thin strips. Wrap 1 slice of bacon around 3 asparagus spears and secure each end with a toothpick. Repeat with the remaining bacon and asparagus.

3. Place the asparagus bundles in the air fryer in a single layer. (If you're using a smaller air fryer, cook in batches if necessary.) Cook for 8 minutes for thin stalks, 10 minutes for medium to thick stalks, or until the asparagus is slightly charred on the ends and the bacon is crispy.

4. Serve with ranch dressing and garnish with chives. Best served fresh. Store leftovers in an airtight container in the fridge for up to 5 days. Reheat in a preheated 400°F air fryer for 3 minutes, or until heated through.

(per serving)   calories **241** | fat **22g** | protein **7g** | total carbs **6g** | fiber **3g**

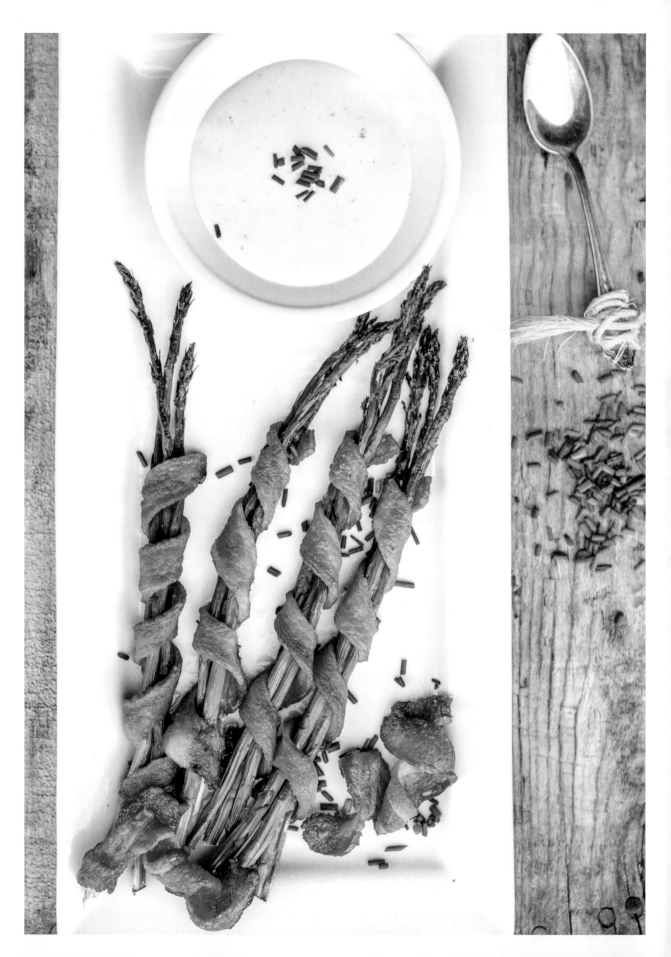

Reuben Egg Rolls

1 (8-ounce) package cream cheese, softened

½ pound cooked corned beef, chopped

½ cup drained and chopped sauerkraut

½ cup shredded Swiss cheese (about 2 ounces)

20 slices prosciutto

THOUSAND ISLAND DIPPING SAUCE:

¾ cup mayonnaise

¼ cup chopped dill pickles

¼ cup tomato sauce

2 tablespoons Swerve confectioners'-style sweetener or equivalent amount of liquid or powdered sweetener (see page 18)

⅛ teaspoon fine sea salt

Fresh thyme leaves, for garnish

Ground black pepper, for garnish

Sauerkraut, for serving (optional)

1. Spray the air fryer basket with avocado oil. Preheat the air fryer to 400°F.

2. Make the filling: Place the cream cheese in a medium-sized bowl and stir to break it up. Add the corned beef, sauerkraut, and Swiss cheese and stir well to combine.

3. Assemble the egg rolls: Lay 1 slice of prosciutto on a sushi mat or a sheet of parchment paper with a short end toward you. Lay another slice of prosciutto on top of it at a right angle, forming a cross. Spoon 3 to 4 tablespoons of the filling into the center of the cross.

4. Fold the sides of the top slice up and over the filling to form the ends of the roll. Tightly roll up the long piece of prosciutto, starting at the edge closest to you, into a tight egg roll shape that overlaps by an inch or so. (Note: If the prosciutto rips, it's okay. It will seal when you fry it.) Repeat with the remaining prosciutto and filling.

5. Place the egg rolls in the air fryer seam side down, leaving space between them. (If you're using a smaller air fryer, cook in batches if necessary.) Cook for 10 minutes, or until the outside is crispy.

6. While the egg rolls are cooking, make the dipping sauce: In a small bowl, combine the mayo, pickles, tomato sauce, sweetener, and salt. Stir well and garnish with thyme and ground black pepper. (The dipping sauce can be made up to 3 days ahead.)

7. Serve the egg rolls with the dipping sauce and sauerkraut if desired. Best served fresh. Store leftovers in an airtight container in the refrigerator for up to 5 days or in the freezer for up to a month. Reheat in a preheated 400°F air fryer for 4 minutes, or until heated through and crispy.

   (per serving)   calories **321** | fat **29g** | protein **13g** | total carbs **1g** | fiber **0.1g**

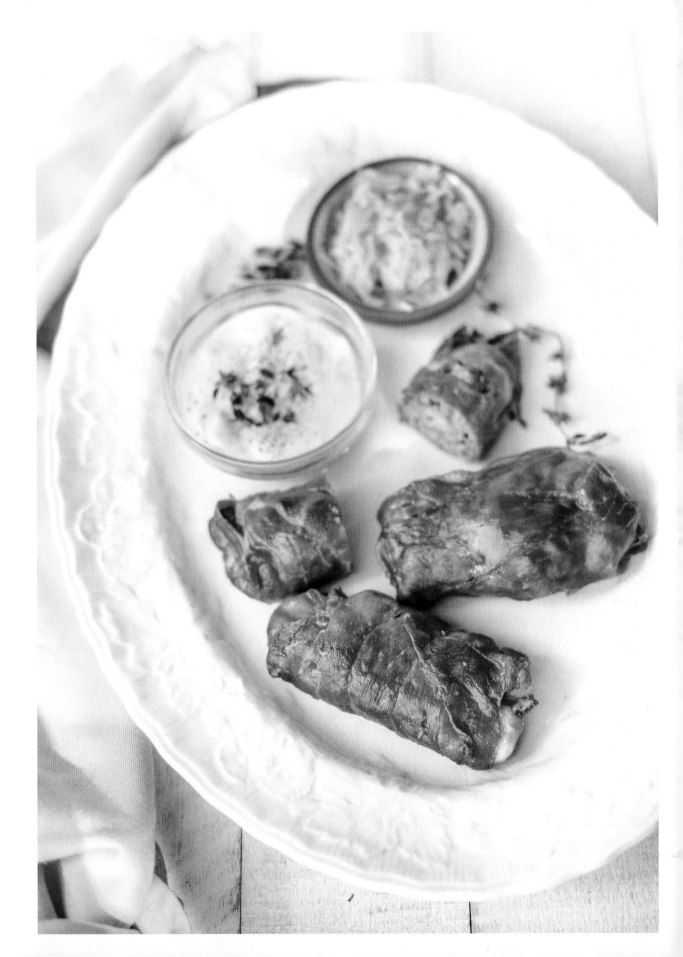

Mozzarella Sticks

yield: 24 mozzarella sticks (2 per serving)
prep time: 15 minutes, plus 2 hours to freeze *cook time:* 14 minutes per batch

DOUGH:

1¾ cups shredded mozzarella cheese (about 7 ounces)

2 tablespoons unsalted butter

1 large egg, beaten

¾ cup blanched almond flour

⅛ teaspoon fine sea salt

24 pieces of string cheese

SPICE MIX:

¼ cup grated Parmesan cheese

3 tablespoons garlic powder

1 tablespoon dried oregano leaves

1 tablespoon onion powder

FOR SERVING (OPTIONAL):

½ cup marinara sauce

½ cup pesto (page 202)

1. Make the dough: Place the mozzarella and butter in a large microwave-safe bowl and microwave for 1 to 2 minutes, until the cheese is entirely melted. Stir well.

2. Add the egg and, using a hand mixer on low, combine well. Add the almond flour and salt and combine well with the mixer.

3. Lay a piece of parchment paper on the countertop and place the dough on it. Knead it for about 3 minutes; the dough should be thick yet pliable. (Note: If the dough is too sticky, chill it in the refrigerator for an hour or overnight.)

4. Scoop up 3 tablespoons of the dough and flatten it into a very thin 3½ by 2-inch rectangle. Place one piece of string cheese in the center and use your hands to press the dough tightly around it. Repeat with the remaining string cheese and dough.

5. In a shallow dish, combine the spice mix ingredients. Place a wrapped piece of string cheese in the dish and roll while pressing down to form a nice crust. Repeat with the remaining pieces of string cheese. Place in the freezer for 2 hours.

6. Ten minutes before air frying, spray the air fryer basket with avocado oil and preheat the air fryer to 425°F.

7. Place the frozen mozzarella sticks in the air fryer basket, leaving space between them, and cook for 9 to 12 minutes, until golden brown. Remove from the air fryer and serve with marinara sauce and pesto, if desired.

8. Store leftovers in an airtight container in the refrigerator for up to 3 days or in the freezer for up to a month. Reheat in a preheated 425°F air fryer for 4 minutes, or until warmed through.

busy family tip: My kids love these so much that I make a triple batch and store extras in the freezer!

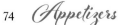
(per serving)   calories **337** | fat **27g** | protein **23g** | total carbs **4g** | fiber **1g**

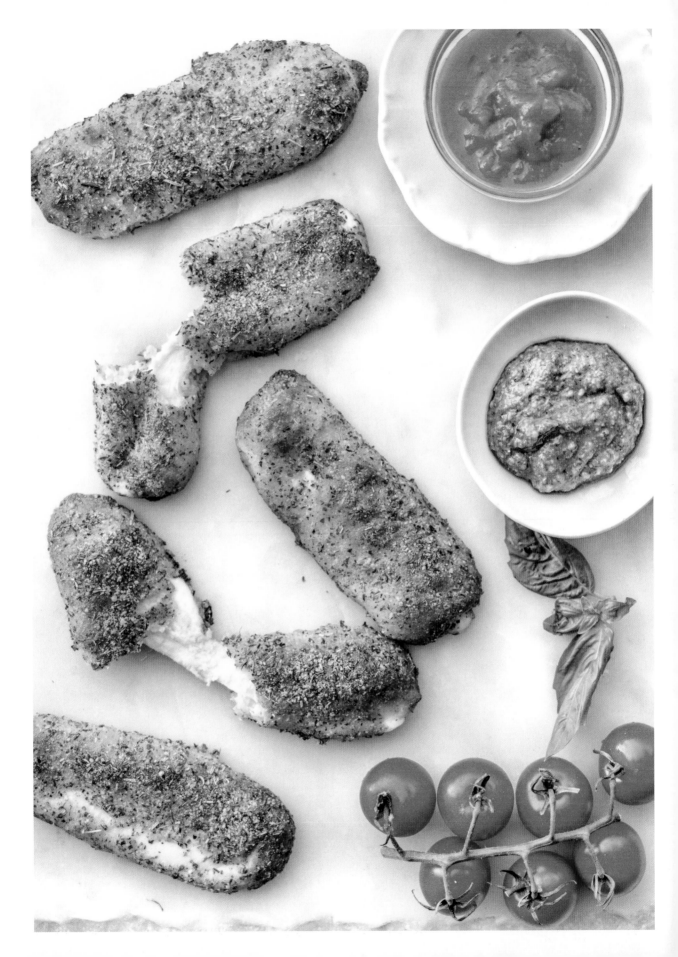

Crispy Calamari Rings

yield: 4 servings   *prep time:* 10 minutes   *cook time:* 15 minutes

option   KETO

2 large egg yolks (see Note)

1 cup powdered Parmesan cheese (see page 19) (or pork dust for dairy-free; see page 19)

¼ cup coconut flour

3 teaspoons dried oregano leaves

½ teaspoon garlic powder

½ teaspoon onion powder

1 pound calamari, sliced into rings (see Tip)

Fresh oregano leaves, for garnish (optional)

1 cup marinara sauce, for serving (optional)

Lemon slices, for serving (optional)

1. Spray the air fryer basket with avocado oil. Preheat the air fryer to 400°F.

2. In a shallow dish, whisk the egg yolks. In a separate bowl, mix together the Parmesan, coconut flour, and spices.

3. Dip the calamari rings in the egg yolks, tap off any excess egg, then dip them into the cheese mixture and coat well. Use your hands to press the coating onto the calamari if necessary. Spray the coated rings with avocado oil.

4. Place the calamari rings in the air fryer, leaving space between them, and cook for 15 minutes, or until golden brown. Garnish with fresh oregano, if desired, and serve with marinara sauce for dipping and lemon slices, if desired.

5. Best served fresh. Store leftovers in an airtight container in the fridge for up to 5 days. Reheat in a preheated 400°F air fryer for 3 minutes, or until heated through.

note: Using only egg yolks helps the coating cling to the calamari rings.

busy family tip: I purchase frozen calamari rings from a local seafood store, which makes this recipe even easier.

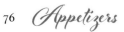

(per serving)   calories **287** | fat **13g** | protein **28g** | total carbs **11g** | fiber **3g**

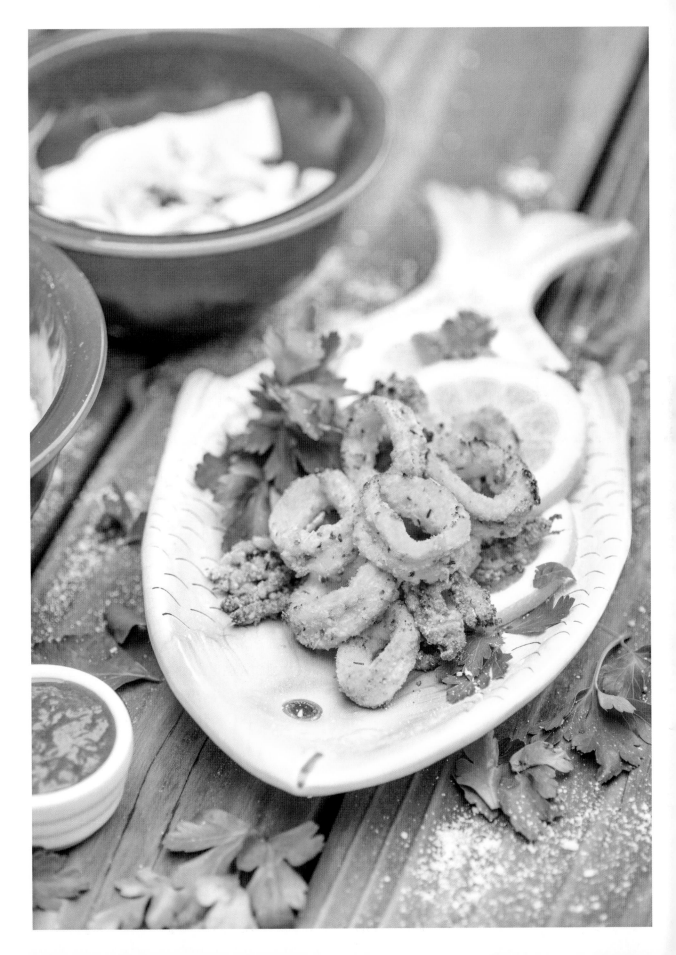

Bloomin' Onion

yield: 8 servings *prep time:* 10 minutes *cook time:* 35 minutes

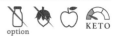

1 extra-large onion (about 3 inches in diameter)

2 large eggs

1 tablespoon water

½ cup powdered Parmesan cheese (about 1½ ounces; see page 19) (or pork dust for dairy-free; see page 19)

2 teaspoons paprika

1 teaspoon garlic powder

¼ teaspoon cayenne pepper

¼ teaspoon fine sea salt

¼ teaspoon ground black pepper

FOR GARNISH (OPTIONAL):

Fresh parsley leaves

Powdered Parmesan cheese (see page 19)

FOR SERVING (OPTIONAL):

Prepared yellow mustard

Ranch Dressing (page 68)

Reduced-sugar or sugar-free ketchup

1. Spray the air fryer basket with avocado oil. Preheat the air fryer to 350°F.

2. Using a sharp knife, cut the top ½ inch off the onion and peel off the outer layer. Cut the onion into 8 equal sections, stopping 1 inch from the bottom—you want the onion to stay together at the base. Gently spread the sections, or "petals," apart.

3. Crack the eggs into a large bowl, add the water, and whisk well. Place the onion in the dish and coat it well in the egg. Use a spoon to coat the inside of the onion and all of the petals.

4. In a small bowl, combine the Parmesan, seasonings, salt, and pepper.

5. Place the onion in a 6-inch pie pan or casserole dish. Sprinkle the seasoning mixture all over the onion and use your fingers to press it into the petals. Spray the onion with avocado oil.

6. Loosely cover the onion with parchment paper and then foil. Place the dish in the air fryer. Cook for 30 minutes, then remove it from the air fryer and increase the air fryer temperature to 400°F.

7. Remove the foil and parchment and spray the onion with avocado oil again. Protecting your hands with oven-safe gloves or a tea towel, transfer the onion to the air fryer basket. Cook for an additional 3 to 5 minutes, until light brown and crispy.

8. Garnish with fresh parsley and powdered Parmesan, if desired. Serve with mustard, ranch dressing, and ketchup, if desired.

9. Store leftovers in an airtight container in the fridge for up to 4 days. Reheat in a preheated 400°F air fryer for 3 to 5 minutes, until warm and crispy.

(per serving) calories **51** | fat **3g** | protein **4g** | total carbs **3g** | fiber **0.4g**

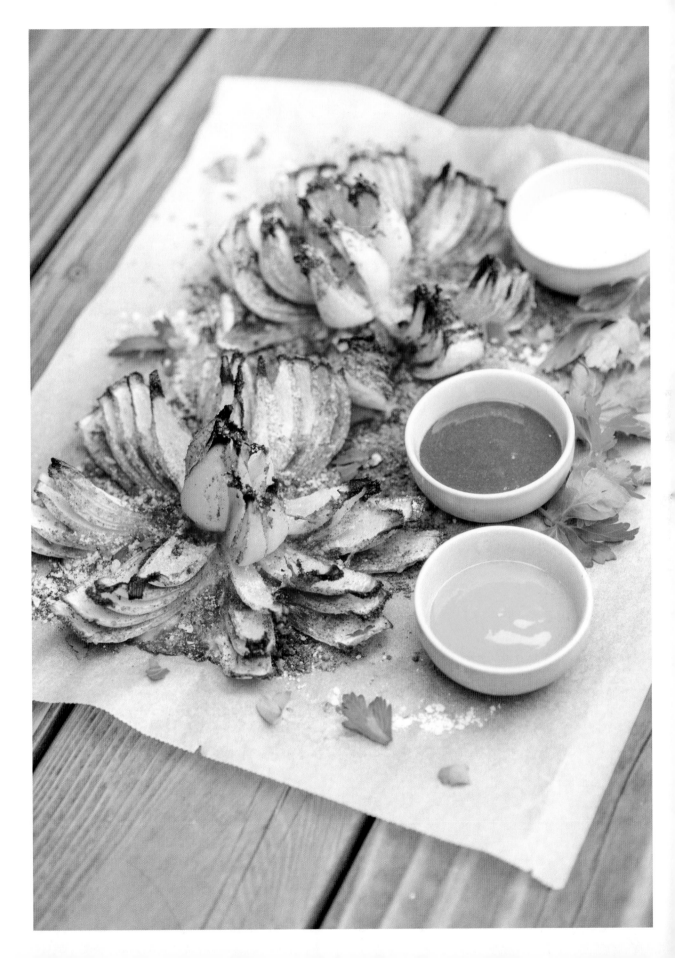

Prosciutto-Wrapped Guacamole Rings

yield: 8 rings (1 per serving) *prep time:* 10 minutes, plus 2 hours to freeze
cook time: 6 minutes

GUACAMOLE:

2 avocados, halved, pitted, and peeled

3 tablespoons lime juice, plus more to taste

2 small plum tomatoes, diced

½ cup finely diced onions

2 small cloves garlic, smashed to a paste

3 tablespoons chopped fresh cilantro leaves

½ scant teaspoon fine sea salt

½ scant teaspoon ground cumin

2 small onions (about 1½ inches in diameter), cut into ½-inch-thick slices

8 slices prosciutto

1. Make the guacamole: Place the avocados and lime juice in a large bowl and mash with a fork until it reaches your desired consistency. Add the tomatoes, onions, garlic, cilantro, salt, and cumin and stir until well combined. Taste and add more lime juice if desired. Set aside half of the guacamole for serving. (Note: If you're making the guacamole ahead of time, place it in a large resealable plastic bag, squeeze out all the air, and seal it shut. It will keep in the refrigerator for up to 3 days when stored this way.)

2. Place a piece of parchment paper on a tray that fits in your freezer and place the onion slices on it, breaking the slices apart into 8 rings. Fill each ring with about 2 tablespoons of guacamole. Place the tray in the freezer for 2 hours.

3. Spray the air fryer basket with avocado oil. Preheat the air fryer to 400°F.

4. Remove the rings from the freezer and wrap each in a slice of prosciutto. Place them in the air fryer basket, leaving space between them (if you're using a smaller air fryer, work in batches if necessary), and cook for 6 minutes, flipping halfway through. Use a spatula to remove the rings from the air fryer. Serve with the reserved half of the guacamole.

5. Store leftovers in an airtight container in the refrigerator for up to 4 days. Reheat in a preheated 400°F air fryer for about 3 minutes, until heated through.

(per serving) calories **132** | fat **9g** | protein **5g** | total carbs **10g** | fiber **4g**

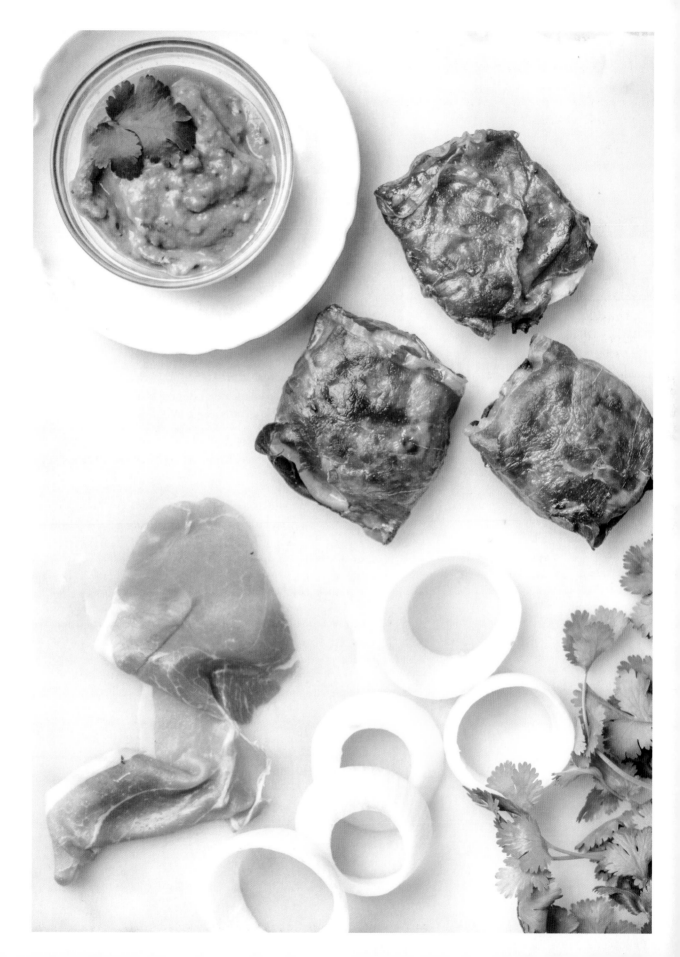

Prosciutto Pierogi

yield: 4 pierogi (1 per serving)   *prep time:* 15 minutes   *cook time:* 20 minutes

1 cup chopped cauliflower

2 tablespoons diced onions

1 tablespoon unsalted butter (or lard or bacon fat for dairy-free), melted

Pinch of fine sea salt

½ cup shredded sharp cheddar cheese (about 2 ounces) (or Kite Hill brand cream cheese style spread, softened, for dairy-free)

8 slices prosciutto

Fresh oregano leaves, for garnish (optional)

1. Preheat the air fryer to 350°F. Lightly grease a 7-inch pie pan or a casserole dish that will fit in your air fryer.

2. Make the filling: Place the cauliflower and onion in the pan. Drizzle with the melted butter and sprinkle with the salt. Using your hands, mix everything together, making sure the cauliflower is coated in the butter.

3. Place the cauliflower mixture in the air fryer and cook for 10 minutes, until fork-tender, stirring halfway through.

4. Transfer the cauliflower mixture to a food processor or high-powered blender. Spray the air fryer basket with avocado oil and increase the air fryer temperature to 400°F.

5. Pulse the cauliflower mixture in the food processor until smooth. Stir in the cheese.

6. Assemble the pierogi: Lay 1 slice of prosciutto on a sheet of parchment paper with a short end toward you. Lay another slice of prosciutto on top of it at a right angle, forming a cross. Spoon about 2 heaping tablespoons of the filling into the center of the cross.

7. Fold each arm of the prosciutto cross over the filling to form a square, making sure that the filling is well covered. Using your fingers, press down around the filling to even out the square shape. Repeat with the rest of the prosciutto and filling.

8. Spray the pierogi with avocado oil and place them in the air fryer basket. Cook for 10 minutes, or until crispy.

9. Garnish with oregano before serving, if desired. Store leftovers in an airtight container in the fridge for up to 4 days. Reheat in a preheated 400°F air fryer for 3 minutes, or until heated through.

(per serving)   calories **150** | fat **11g** | protein **11g** | total carbs **2g** | fiber **1g**

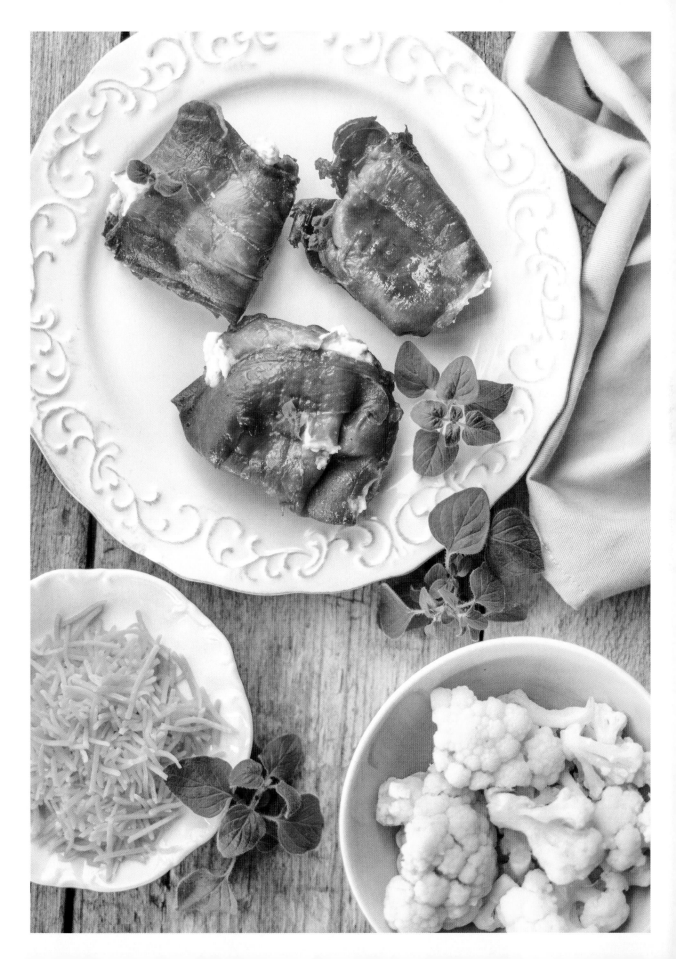

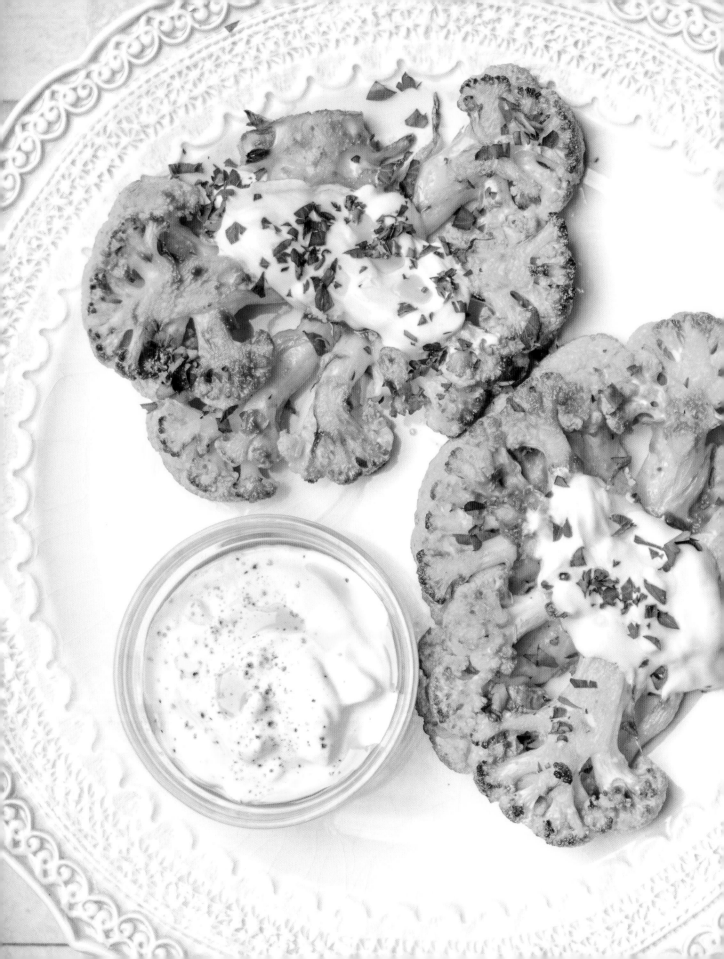

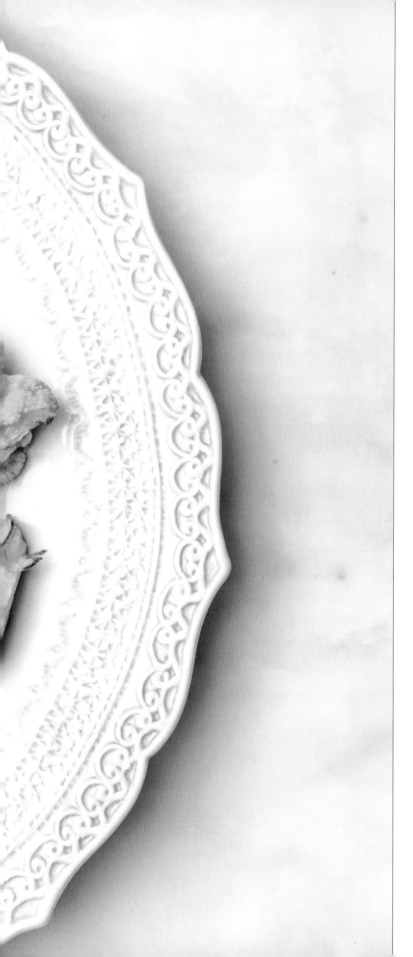

Sides and Vegetarian

Keto Tots

yield: 6 servings   *prep time:* 10 minutes   *cook time:* 15 minutes

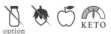

3 cups cauliflower florets

1 tablespoon coconut flour

1 teaspoon fine sea salt

1 large egg, beaten

1 (8-ounce) package cream cheese (or Kite Hill brand cream cheese style spread for dairy-free), softened

½ cup finely chopped onions

1 teaspoon smoked paprika

Chopped fresh parsley, for garnish (optional)

Ranch Dressing (page 68), for serving (optional)

1. Spray the air fryer basket with avocado oil. Preheat the air fryer to 400°F.

2. Place the cauliflower in a food processor and pulse until it resembles grains of rice.

3. Place the riced cauliflower in a medium-sized bowl, sprinkle the coconut flour and salt on top, and toss well to coat. Add the egg, cream cheese, onions, and paprika and mix well to combine.

4. Form the cauliflower–cream cheese mixture into 24 tater tot shapes. Place them in the air fryer basket, leaving space between them, and cook for 15 minutes, or until golden brown.

5. Remove the tots from the air fryer and place them on a serving plate. Garnish with chopped fresh parsley, if desired, and serve with ranch dressing on the side for dipping, if desired.

6. Store leftovers in an airtight container in the fridge for 3 days or in the freezer for up to a month. Reheat in a preheated 400°F air fryer for 4 minutes, or until heated through.

(per serving)   calories **166** | fat **13g** | protein **5g** | total carbs **5g** | fiber **2g**

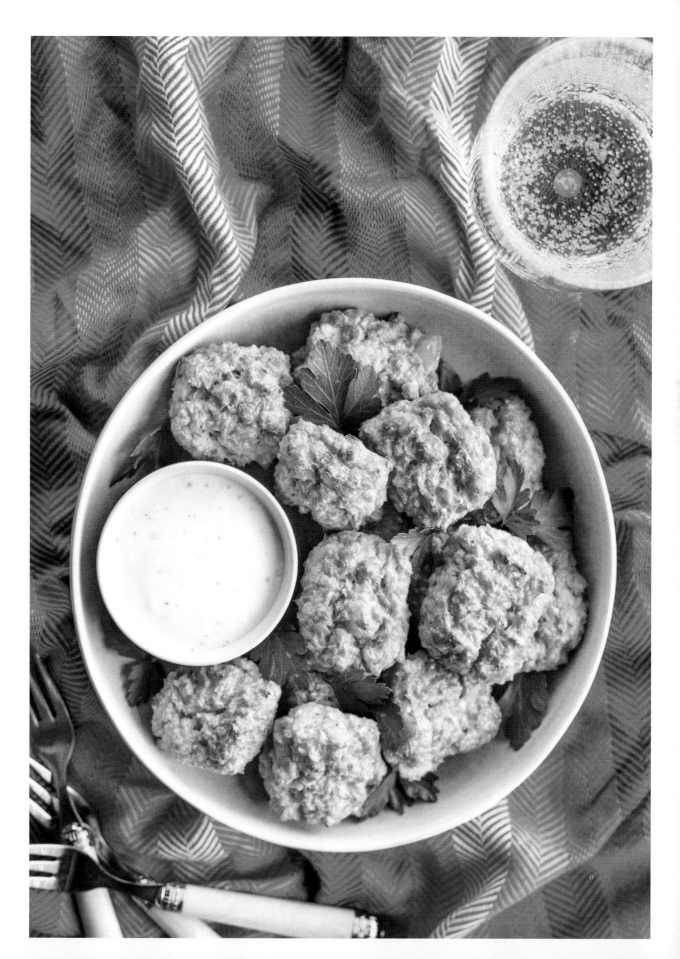

Loaded Bacon-Wrapped Keto Tots

yield: 6 servings *prep time:* 10 minutes *cook time:* 13 minutes

1 recipe Keto Tots (page 86)

12 thin-cut slices bacon, cut in half crosswise

½ cup shredded cheddar cheese (about 2 ounces)

¼ cup sliced green onions, for garnish

½ cup full-fat sour cream, for serving

1. Spray the air fryer basket with avocado oil. Preheat the air fryer to 400°F.

2. Wrap a piece of bacon around each tot and secure it with a toothpick. Place the wrapped tots in the air fryer basket, leaving space between them.

3. Cook for 10 to 13 minutes, until the bacon is crisp to your liking. Remove the tots from the air fryer, place them on a serving plate, and sprinkle the cheese over the hot tots. Garnish with the green onions and serve with the sour cream.

4. If you're making these in advance, store the cooked bacon-wrapped tots separately from the cheese in an airtight container in the fridge for up to 4 days or in the freezer for up to a month. Reheat in a preheated 400°F air fryer for 5 minutes, or until crisp to your liking, and top with the cheese as instructed.

(per serving) calories **385** | fat **31g** | protein **16g** | total carbs **6g** | fiber **2g**

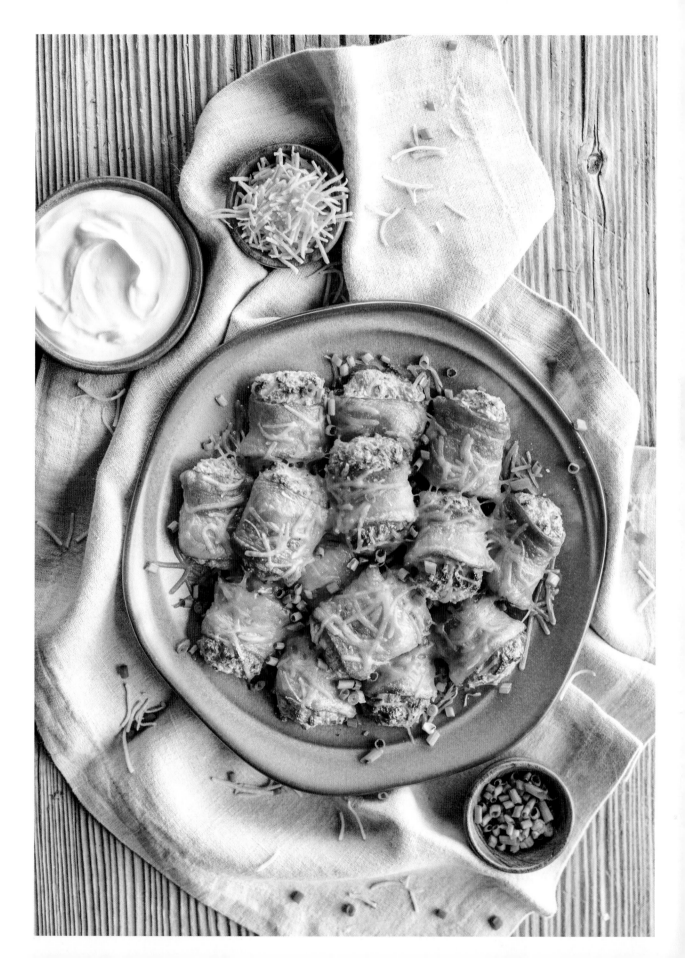

Tomatoes Provençal

yield: 4 servings   *prep time:* 10 minutes   *cook time:* 15 minutes

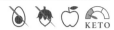

4 small ripe tomatoes connected on the vine

¼ teaspoon fine sea salt

¼ teaspoon ground black pepper

½ cup powdered Parmesan cheese (about 1½ ounces) (see page 19)

2 tablespoons chopped fresh parsley

¼ cup minced onions

2 cloves garlic, minced

½ teaspoon chopped fresh thyme leaves

FOR GARNISH:

Fresh parsley leaves

Ground black pepper

Sprig of fresh basil

1. Spray the air fryer basket with avocado oil. Preheat the air fryer to 350°F.

2. Slice the tops off the tomatoes without removing them from the vine. Do not discard the tops. Use a large spoon to scoop the seeds out of the tomatoes. Sprinkle the insides of the tomatoes with the salt and pepper.

3. In a medium-sized bowl, combine the cheese, parsley, onions, garlic, and thyme. Stir to combine well. Divide the mixture evenly among the tomatoes.

4. Spray avocado oil on the tomatoes and place them in the air fryer basket. Place the tomato tops in the air fryer basket next to, not on top of, the filled tomatoes. Cook for 15 minutes, or until the filling is golden and the tomatoes are soft yet still holding their shape.

5. Garnish with fresh parsley, ground black pepper, and a sprig of basil. Serve warm, with the tomato tops on the vine.

6. Store leftovers in an airtight container in the refrigerator for up to 4 days. Reheat in a preheated 350°F air fryer for about 3 minutes, until heated through.

busy family tip: If you're short on time or don't have tomatoes on the vine, you can use 2 large ripe tomatoes instead, sliced in half crosswise to form 4 tomato halves.

(per serving)   calories **68** | fat **3g** | protein **5g** | total carbs **6g** | fiber **1g**

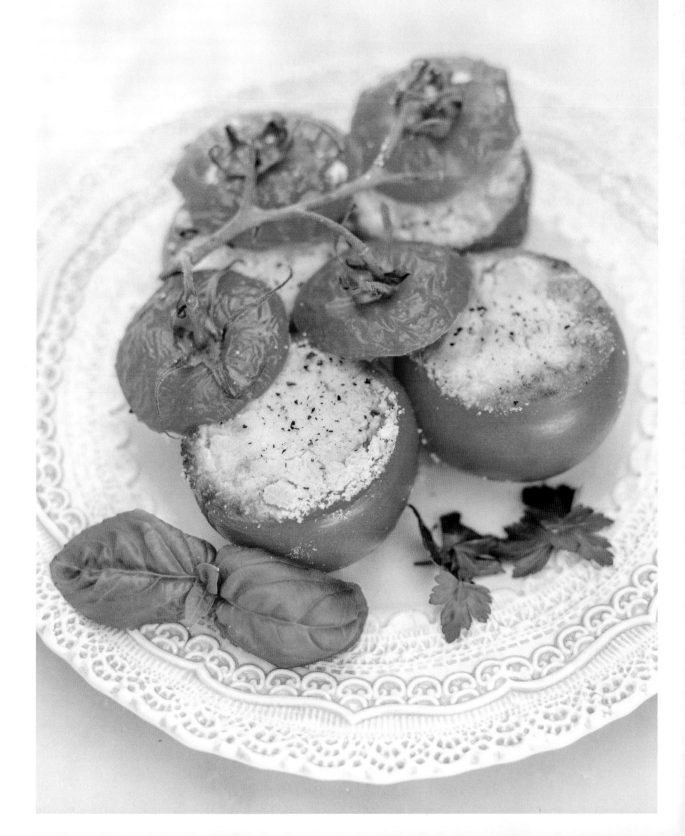

Burrata-Stuffed Tomatoes

yield: 4 servings   *prep time:* 5 minutes   *cook time:* 5 minutes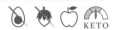

4 medium tomatoes

½ teaspoon fine sea salt

4 (2-ounce) Burrata balls

Fresh basil leaves, for garnish

Extra-virgin olive oil, for drizzling

1. Preheat the air fryer to 300°F.

2. Core the tomatoes and scoop out the seeds and membranes using a melon baller or spoon. Sprinkle the insides of the tomatoes with the salt.

3. Stuff each tomato with a ball of Burrata. Place in the air fryer and cook for 5 minutes, or until the cheese has softened.

4. Garnish with basil leaves and drizzle with olive oil. Serve warm.

5. Store leftovers in an airtight container in the refrigerator for up to 4 days. Reheat in a preheated 300°F air fryer for about 3 minutes, until heated through.

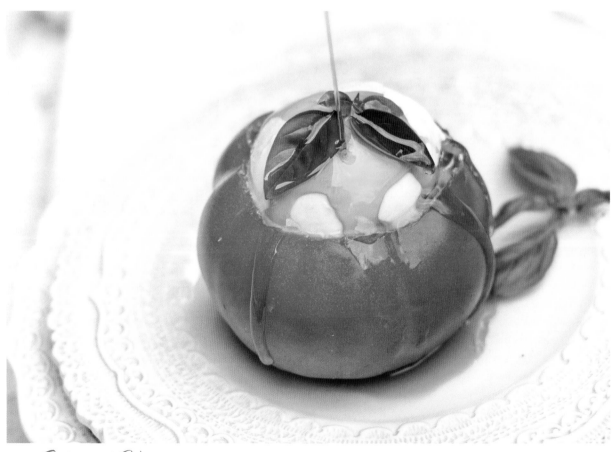

Sides and Vegetarian   (per serving)   calories **108** | fat **7g** | protein **6g** | total carbs **5g** | fiber **2g**

Crispy Brussels Sprouts

yield: 4 servings   *prep time:* 5 minutes   *cook time:* 8 minutes

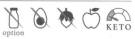

2 cups Brussels sprouts, trimmed and halved

3 tablespoons ghee or coconut oil, melted

1 teaspoon fine sea salt or smoked salt

Dash of lime or lemon juice

Thinly sliced Parmesan cheese, for serving (optional; omit for dairy-free)

Lemon slices, for serving (optional)

1. Spray the air fryer basket with avocado oil. Preheat the air fryer to 400°F.

2. In a large bowl, toss together the Brussels sprouts, ghee, and salt. Add the lime or lemon juice.

3. Place the Brussels sprouts in the air fryer basket and cook for 8 minutes, or until crispy, shaking the basket after 5 minutes. Serve with thinly sliced Parmesan and lemon slices, if desired.

4. Best served fresh. Store leftovers in an airtight container in the fridge for up to 5 days. Reheat in a preheated 390°F air fryer for 3 minutes, or until heated through.

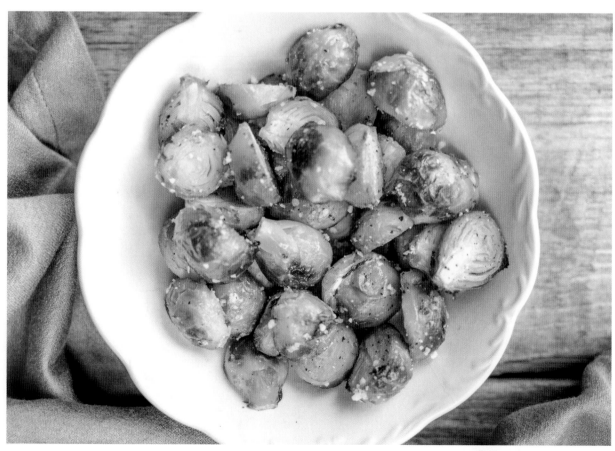

(per serving)   calories **149** | fat **12g** | protein **4g** | total carbs **10g** | fiber **4g**

Caramelized Broccoli

yield: 4 servings   *prep time:* 5 minutes   *cook time:* 8 minutes

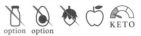

4 cups broccoli florets

3 tablespoons melted ghee or butter-flavored coconut oil

1½ teaspoons fine sea salt or smoked salt

Mayonnaise, for serving (optional; omit for egg-free)

1. Spray the air fryer basket with avocado oil. Preheat the air fryer to 400°F.

2. Place the broccoli in a large bowl. Drizzle it with the ghee, toss to coat, and sprinkle it with the salt. Transfer the broccoli to the air fryer basket and cook for 8 minutes, or until tender and crisp on the edges.

3. Store leftovers in an airtight container in the fridge for up to 4 days or in the freezer for up to a month. Reheat in a preheated 400°F air fryer for 5 minutes, or until crisp.

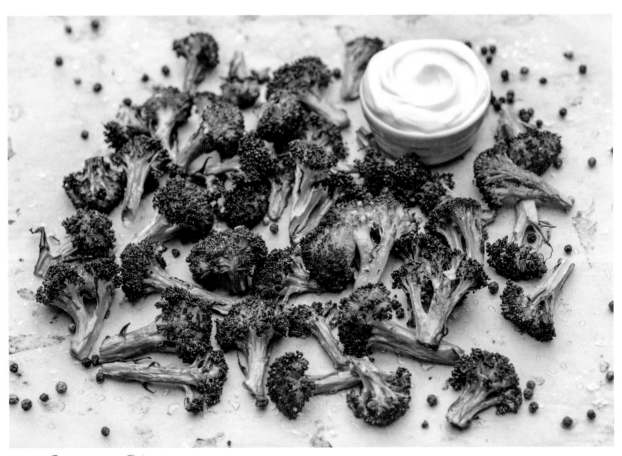

(per serving)   calories **107** | fat **9g** | protein **3g** | total carbs **6g** | fiber **2g**

Perfect Zoodles

yield: 2 servings   *prep time:* 5 minutes   *cook time:* 8 minutes

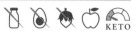

1 (12-inch) zucchini

special equipment:

Spiral slicer

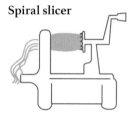

1. Spray the air fryer basket with avocado oil. Preheat the air fryer to 400°F.

2. Cut the ends off the zucchini to create nice even edges. If you desire completely white noodles, peel the zucchini. Using a spiral slicer, cut the zucchini into long, thin noodles.

3. Spread out the zucchini noodles in the air fryer basket in a single layer and cook for 8 minutes, or until soft. Remove from the air fryer and serve immediately.

4. Store leftovers in an airtight container for 4 days. Reheat in a single layer in the air fryer for 3 minutes, or until heated through.

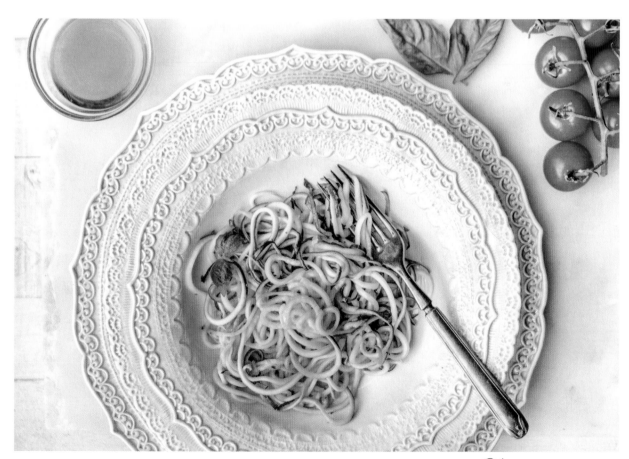

(per serving)   calories **29** | fat **0g** | protein **2g** | total carbs **6g** | fiber **2g**

Marinated Turmeric Cauliflower Steaks

yield: 4 servings *prep time:* 5 minutes, plus 20 minutes to marinate *cook time:* 15 minutes

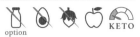

¼ cup avocado oil

¼ cup lemon juice

2 cloves garlic, minced

1 teaspoon grated fresh ginger

1 tablespoon turmeric powder

1 teaspoon fine sea salt

1 medium head cauliflower

Full-fat sour cream (or Kite Hill brand almond milk yogurt for dairy-free), for serving (optional)

Extra-virgin olive oil, for serving (optional)

Chopped fresh cilantro leaves, for garnish (optional)

1. Preheat the air fryer to 400°F.

2. In a large shallow dish, combine the avocado oil, lemon juice, garlic, ginger, turmeric, and salt. Slice the cauliflower into ½-inch steaks and place them in the marinade. Cover and refrigerate for 20 minutes or overnight.

3. Remove the cauliflower steaks from the marinade and place them in the air fryer basket. Cook for 15 minutes, or until tender and slightly charred on the edges.

4. Serve with sour cream and a drizzle of olive oil, and sprinkle with chopped cilantro leaves if desired.

5. Store leftovers in an airtight container in the fridge for up to 4 days or in the freezer for up to a month. Reheat in a preheated 400°F air fryer for 5 minutes, or until warm.

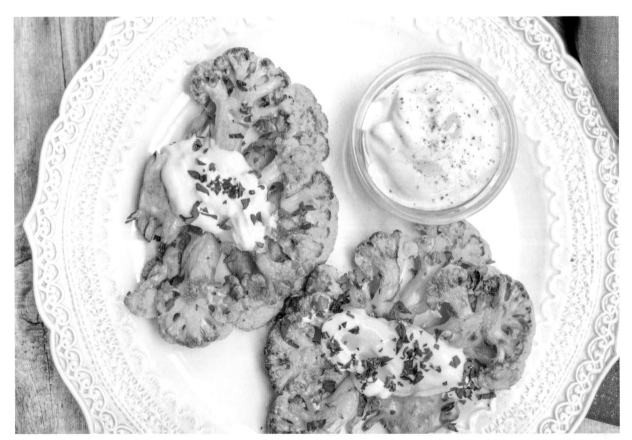

(per serving) calories **69** | fat **4g** | protein **4g** | total carbs **8g** | fiber **4g**

Caramelized Ranch Cauliflower

yield: 4 servings   *prep time:* 5 minutes   *cook time:* 12 minutes

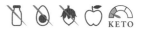

4 cups cauliflower florets

2 tablespoons dried parsley

1 tablespoon plus 1 teaspoon onion powder

2 teaspoons garlic powder

1½ teaspoons dried dill weed

1 teaspoon dried chives

1 teaspoon fine sea salt or smoked salt

1 teaspoon ground black pepper

Ranch Dressing (page 68), for serving (optional)

1. Preheat the air fryer to 400°F.

2. Place the cauliflower in a large bowl and spray it with avocado oil.

3. Place the parsley, onion powder, garlic powder, dill weed, chives, salt, and pepper in a small bowl and stir to combine well. Sprinkle the ranch seasoning over the cauliflower.

4. Place the cauliflower in the air fryer and cook for 12 minutes, or until tender and crisp on the edges. Serve with ranch dressing for dipping, if desired.

5. Store leftovers in an airtight container in the fridge for up to 4 days or in the freezer for up to a month. Reheat in a preheated 400°F air fryer for 5 minutes, or until crisp.

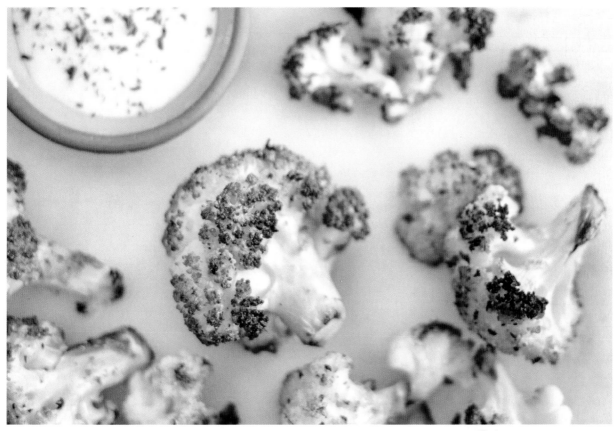

(per serving)   calories **62** | fat **0.1g** | protein **6g** | total carbs **12g** | fiber **6g**

Fried Cauliflower Rice

yield: 4 servings   *prep time:* 5 minutes   *cook time:* 8 minutes

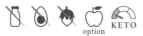

2 cups cauliflower florets

⅓ cup sliced green onions, plus more for garnish

3 tablespoons wheat-free tamari or coconut aminos

1 clove garlic, smashed to a paste or minced

1 teaspoon grated fresh ginger

1 teaspoon fish sauce or fine sea salt (see Note)

1 teaspoon lime juice

⅛ teaspoon ground black pepper

note: One staple that every cook should have in the refrigerator is fish sauce, which takes food from good to amazing. Its secret? The umami flavor. Like saltiness and sweetness, umami is a category of taste, and it's savory, satisfying, and meaty. Red Boat brand fish sauce is traditionally fermented and does not contain wheat like other brands.

1. Preheat the air fryer to 375°F.

2. Place the cauliflower in a food processor and pulse until it resembles grains of rice.

3. Place all the ingredients, including the riced cauliflower, in a large bowl and stir well to combine.

4. Transfer the cauliflower mixture to a 6-inch pie pan or a casserole dish that will fit in your air fryer. Cook for 8 minutes, or until soft, shaking halfway through. Garnish with sliced green onions before serving.

5. Store leftovers in an airtight container in the fridge for up to 4 days. Reheat in a preheated 375°F air fryer for 4 minutes, or until heated through.

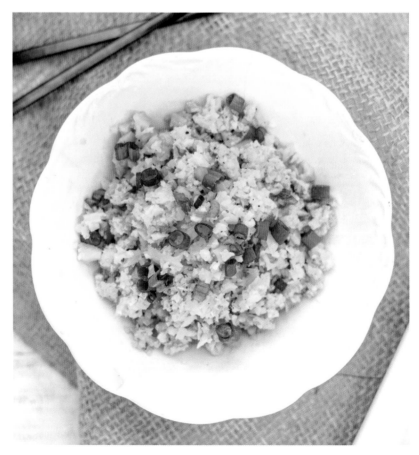

(per serving) calories **30** | fat **0g** | protein **3g** | total carbs **4g** | fiber **1g**

Garlic Thyme Mushrooms

yield: 4 servings *prep time:* 5 minutes *cook time:* 10 minutes

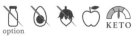

3 tablespoons unsalted butter (or butter-flavored coconut oil for dairy-free), melted

1 (8-ounce) package button mushrooms, sliced

2 cloves garlic, minced

3 sprigs fresh thyme leaves, plus more for garnish

½ teaspoon fine sea salt

tip: These tasty mushrooms are great on steak, chicken, or burgers!

1. Spray the air fryer basket with avocado oil. Preheat the air fryer to 400°F.

2. Place all the ingredients in a medium-sized bowl. Use a spoon or your hands to coat the mushroom slices.

3. Place the mushrooms in the air fryer basket in one layer; work in batches if necessary. Cook for 10 minutes, or until slightly crispy and brown. Garnish with thyme sprigs before serving.

4. Store leftovers in an airtight container in the fridge for up to 5 days or in the freezer for up to a month. Reheat in a preheated 350°F air fryer for 5 minutes, or until heated through.

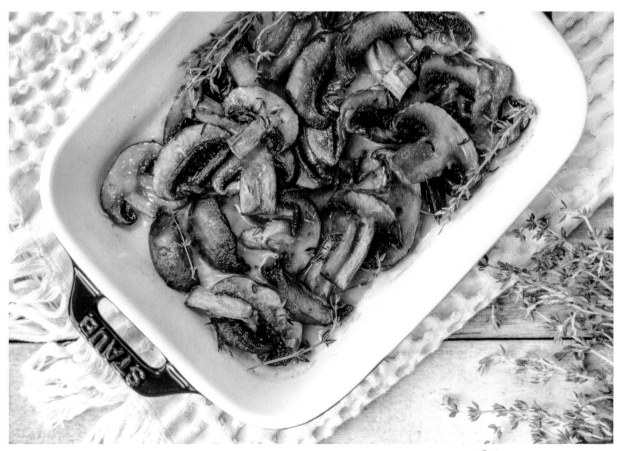

(per serving) calories **82** | fat **9g** | protein **1g** | total carbs **1g** | fiber **0.2g**

Sweet Fauxtato Casserole

yield: 6 servings   *prep time:* 15 minutes   *cook time:* 55 minutes

2 cups cauliflower florets (see Tip)

1 cup chicken broth or water

1 cup canned pumpkin puree

⅓ cup unsalted butter, melted (or coconut oil for dairy-free), plus more for the pan

¼ cup Swerve confectioners'-style sweetener or equivalent amount of liquid or powdered sweetener (see page 18)

¼ cup unsweetened, unflavored almond milk or heavy cream

2 large eggs, beaten

1 teaspoon fine sea salt

1 teaspoon vanilla extract

TOPPING:

1 cup chopped pecans

½ cup blanched almond flour or pecan meal

½ cup Swerve confectioners'-style sweetener or equivalent amount of powdered sweetener (see page 18)

⅓ cup unsalted butter, melted (or coconut oil for dairy-free)

Chopped fresh parsley leaves, for garnish (optional)

1. Preheat the air fryer to 350°F.

2. Place the cauliflower florets in a 6-inch pie pan or a casserole dish that will fit in your air fryer. Add the broth to the pie pan. Cook in the air fryer for 20 minutes, or until the cauliflower is very tender.

3. Drain the cauliflower and transfer it to a food processor. Set the pie pan aside; you'll use it in the next step. Blend the cauliflower until very smooth. Add the pumpkin, butter, sweetener, almond milk, eggs, salt, and vanilla and puree until smooth.

4. Grease the pie pan that you cooked the cauliflower in with butter. Pour the cauliflower-pumpkin mixture into the pan. Set aside.

5. Make the topping: In a large bowl, mix together all the ingredients for the topping until well combined. Crumble the topping over the cauliflower-pumpkin mixture.

6. Cook in the air fryer for 30 to 35 minutes, until cooked through and golden brown on top. Garnish with fresh parsley before serving, if desired.

7. Store leftovers in an airtight container in the fridge for up to 4 days or in the freezer for up to a month. Reheat in a preheated 350°F air fryer for 6 minutes, or until heated through.

busy family tip: To make this dish even easier, follow the lead of one of my recipe testers and use 2 cups frozen mashed cauliflower, thawed, in place of the florets. This lets you skip step 2 and go straight to the food processor, so it's much faster! Just make sure the mashed cauliflower is completely thawed before you start.

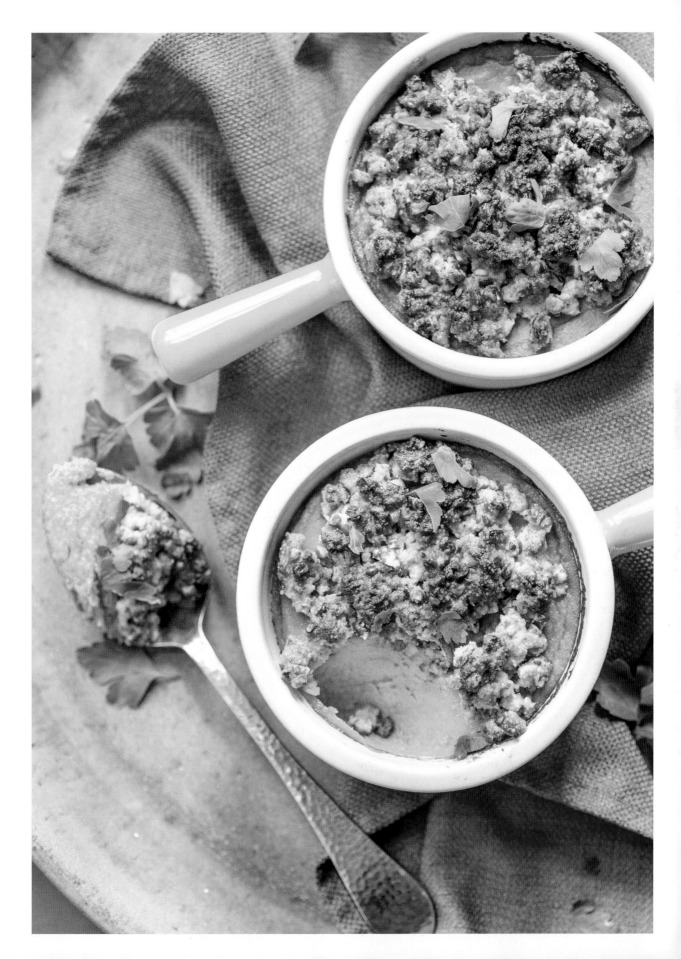

Spinach Artichoke Tart

yield: one 6-inch tart (6 servings)   *prep time:* 10 minutes   *cook time:* 40 minutes

KETO

CRUST:

1 cup blanched almond flour

1 cup grated Parmesan cheese (about 3 ounces)

1 large egg

FILLING:

4 ounces cream cheese (½ cup), softened

1 (8-ounce) package frozen chopped spinach, thawed and drained

½ cup artichoke hearts, drained and chopped

⅓ cup shredded Parmesan cheese, plus more for topping

1 large egg

1 clove garlic, minced

¼ teaspoon fine sea salt

1. Preheat the air fryer to 350°F.

2. Make the crust: Place the almond flour and cheese in a large bowl and mix until well combined. Add the egg and mix until the dough is well combined and stiff.

3. Press the dough into a 6-inch pie pan. Bake for 8 to 10 minutes, until it starts to brown lightly.

4. Meanwhile, make the filling: Place the cream cheese in a large bowl and stir to break it up. Add the spinach, artichoke hearts, cheese, egg, garlic, and salt. Stir well to combine.

5. Pour the spinach mixture into the prebaked crust and sprinkle with additional Parmesan. Place in the air fryer and cook for 25 to 30 minutes, until cooked through.

6. Store leftovers in an airtight container in the fridge for up to 4 days or in the freezer for up to a month. Reheat in a preheated 350°F air fryer for 5 minutes, or until heated through.

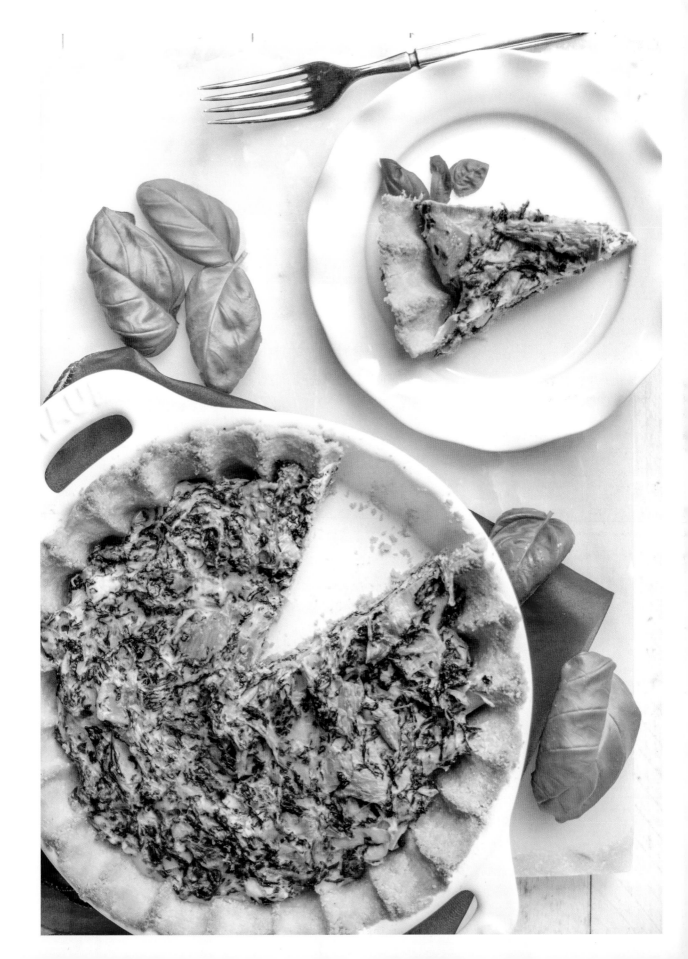

Crunchy-Top Personal Mac 'n' Cheese

yield: 4 servings   *prep time:* 10 minutes   *cook time:* 15 minutes

2 cups frozen chopped cauliflower, thawed

2 ounces cream cheese (¼ cup), softened

¼ cup shredded Gruyère or Swiss cheese

¼ cup shredded sharp cheddar cheese

2 tablespoons finely diced onions

3 tablespoons beef broth

¼ teaspoon fine sea salt

TOPPING:

¼ cup pork dust (see page 19)

¼ cup unsalted butter, melted, plus more for greasing ramekins

4 slices bacon, finely diced

FOR GARNISH (OPTIONAL):

Chopped fresh thyme or chives

1. Preheat the air fryer to 375°F.

2. Place the cauliflower on a paper towel and pat dry. Cut any large pieces of cauliflower into ½-inch pieces.

3. In a medium-sized bowl, stir together the cream cheese, Gruyère, cheddar, and onions. Slowly stir in the broth and combine well. Add the salt and stir to combine. Add the cauliflower and stir gently to mix the cauliflower into the cheese sauce.

4. Grease four 4-ounce ramekins with butter. Divide the cauliflower mixture among the ramekins, filling each three-quarters full.

5. Make the topping: In a small bowl, stir together the pork dust, butter, and bacon until well combined. Divide the topping among the ramekins.

6. Place the ramekins in the air fryer (if you're using a smaller air fryer, work in batches if necessary) and cook for 15 minutes, or until the topping is browned and the bacon is crispy.

7. Garnish with fresh thyme or chives, if desired.

8. Store leftovers in the ramekins covered with foil. Reheat in a preheated 375°F air fryer for 6 minutes, or until the cauliflower is heated through and the top is crispy.

(per serving)   calories **305** | fat **26g** | protein **12g** | total carbs **6g** | fiber **3g**

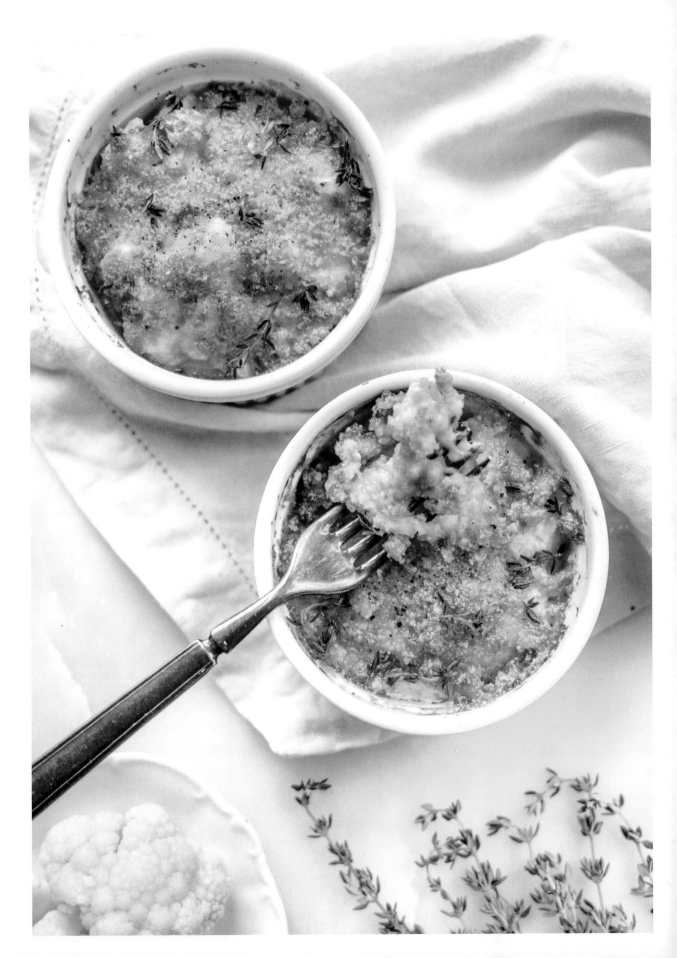

Parmesan Flan

yield: 4 servings   *prep time:* 10 minutes, plus 15 minutes to rest   *cook time:* 25 minutes

½ cup grated Parmesan cheese (about 1½ ounces)

1 cup heavy cream, very warm

⅛ teaspoon fine sea salt

⅛ teaspoon ground white pepper

1 large egg

1 large egg yolk

FOR SERVING/GARNISH (OPTIONAL):

2 cups arugula

1 cup heirloom cherry tomatoes, halved

4 slices Italian cured beef (omit for vegetarian)

Ground black pepper

1. Preheat the air fryer to 350°F. Grease four 4-ounce ramekins well.

2. Place the Parmesan in a medium-sized bowl and pour in the warm cream. Stir well to combine and add the salt and pepper.

3. In a separate medium-sized bowl, beat the egg and yolk until well combined. Gradually stir in the warm Parmesan mixture.

4. Pour the egg-and-cheese mixture into the prepared ramekins, cover the ramekins with foil, and place them in a casserole dish that will fit in your air fryer.

5. Pour boiling water into the casserole dish until the water reaches halfway up the sides of the ramekins. Place the casserole dish in the air fryer and bake until the flan is just set (the mixture will jiggle slightly when moved), about 25 minutes. Check after 20 minutes.

6. Let the flan rest for 15 minutes. Serve with arugula, halved cherry tomatoes, and slices of Italian cured beef, if desired. Garnish with ground black pepper, if desired.

7. Store leftovers in an airtight container in the fridge for up to 5 days. Reheat the flan in a ramekin in a preheated 350°F air fryer for 5 minutes, or until heated through.

(per serving)   calories **345** | fat **32g** | protein **14g** | total carbs **2g** | fiber **0.2g**

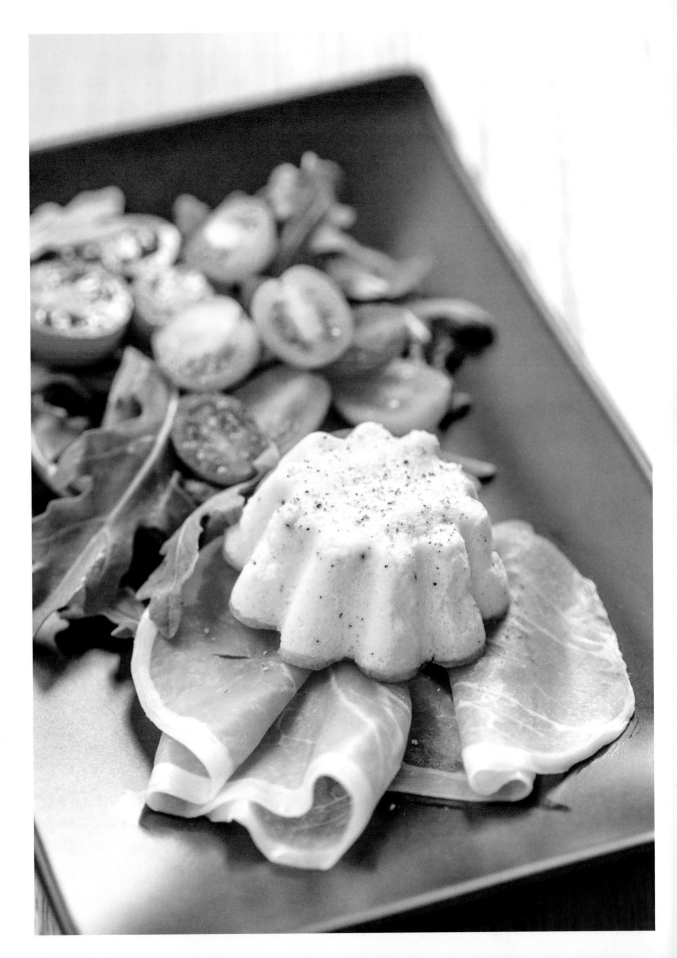

Garlic Butter Breadsticks

yield: 6 breadsticks (1 per serving)   *prep time:* 10 minutes   *cook time:* 12 minutes

KETO

DOUGH:

1¾ cups shredded mozzarella cheese (about 7 ounces)

2 tablespoons unsalted butter

1 large egg, beaten

¾ cup blanched almond flour

⅛ teaspoon fine sea salt

GARLIC BUTTER:

3 tablespoons unsalted butter, softened

2 cloves garlic, minced

TOPPING:

½ cup shredded Parmesan cheese (about 2 ounces)

1 teaspoon dried basil leaves

1 teaspoon dried oregano leaves

FOR SERVING (OPTIONAL):

½ cup marinara sauce

1. Preheat the air fryer to 400°F. Place a piece of parchment paper in a 6-inch square casserole dish and spray it with avocado oil.

2. Make the dough: Place the mozzarella cheese and butter in a microwave-safe bowl and microwave for 1 to 2 minutes, until the cheese is entirely melted. Stir well. Add the egg and, using a hand mixer on low speed, combine well. Add the almond flour and salt and combine well with the hand mixer.

3. Lay a piece of parchment paper on the countertop and place the dough on it. Knead it for about 3 minutes; the dough should be thick yet pliable. (Note: If the dough is too sticky, chill it in the refrigerator for an hour or overnight.) Place the dough in the prepared casserole dish and use your hands to spread it out to fill the bottom of the casserole dish.

4. Make the garlic butter: In a small dish, stir together the butter and garlic until well combined.

5. Spread the garlic butter on top of the dough. Top with the Parmesan, basil, and oregano. Place in the air fryer and cook for 10 minutes, or until golden brown and cooked through.

6. Cut into 1-inch-wide breadsticks and serve with marinara sauce, if desired. Best served fresh, but leftovers can be stored in an airtight container in the fridge for up to 3 days. Reheat in a preheated 400°F air fryer for 3 minutes, or until the cheese is hot and bubbly.

busy family tip: When I make this dish, I quadruple the recipe and store the extra dough in the fridge for up to 4 days or in the freezer for up to a month.

(per serving)   calories **301** | fat **26g** | protein **14g** | total carbs **6g** | fiber **2g**

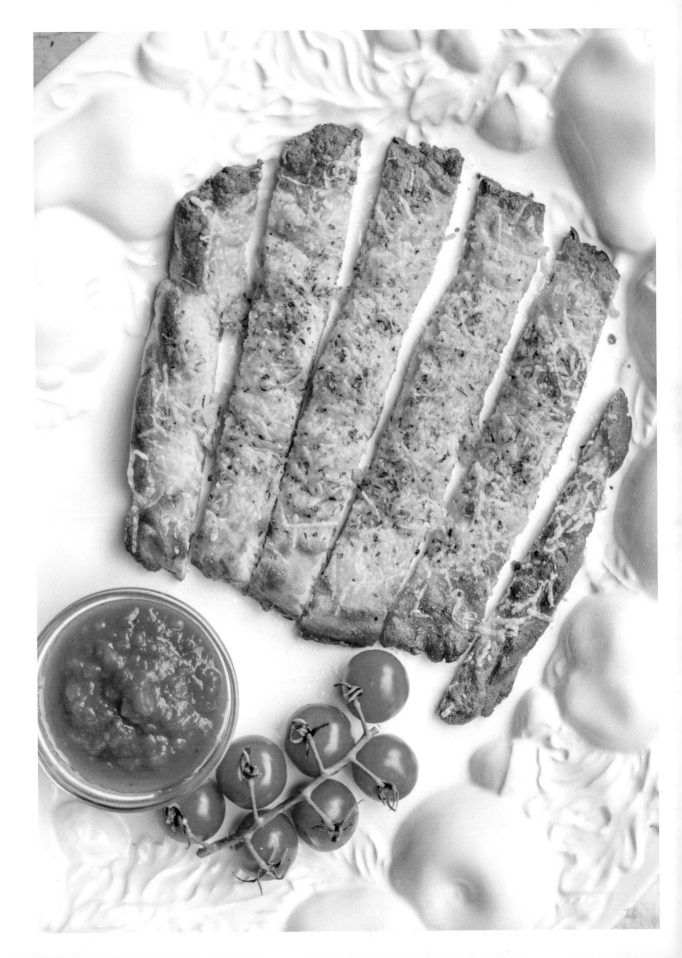

Bruschetta

yield: 12 slices (2 per serving)   *prep time:* 6 minutes   *cook time:* 8 minutes

1 small tomato, diced

2 tablespoons chopped fresh basil leaves

1 teaspoon dried oregano leaves

¼ teaspoon fine sea salt

3 tablespoons unsalted butter, softened (or olive oil for dairy-free)

1 clove garlic, minced

1 recipe Hot Dog Buns (page 226), cut into twelve ½-inch-thick slices

¼ cup plus 2 tablespoons shredded Parmesan cheese

1. Spray the air fryer basket with avocado oil. Preheat the air fryer to 360°F.

2. In a small bowl, stir together the tomato, basil, oregano, and salt until well combined. Set aside.

3. In another small bowl, mix together the butter and garlic. Spread the garlic butter on one side of each hot dog bun slice.

4. Place the slices in the air fryer basket buttered side down, spaced about ⅛ inch apart. Cook for 4 minutes. Remove the slices from the air fryer, flip them so that the buttered side is up, and top each slice with 1½ tablespoons of Parmesan and a dollop of the tomato mixture.

5. Increase the air fryer temperature to 390°F and return the slices to the air fryer basket. Cook for another 2 to 4 minutes, until the bread is crispy and the cheese is melted.

6. Serve immediately. Alternatively, stop after step 3 and store the slices of bread and the tomato mixture in separate airtight containers in the fridge for up to 5 days. When you're ready to eat, cook as instructed in steps 4 and 5.

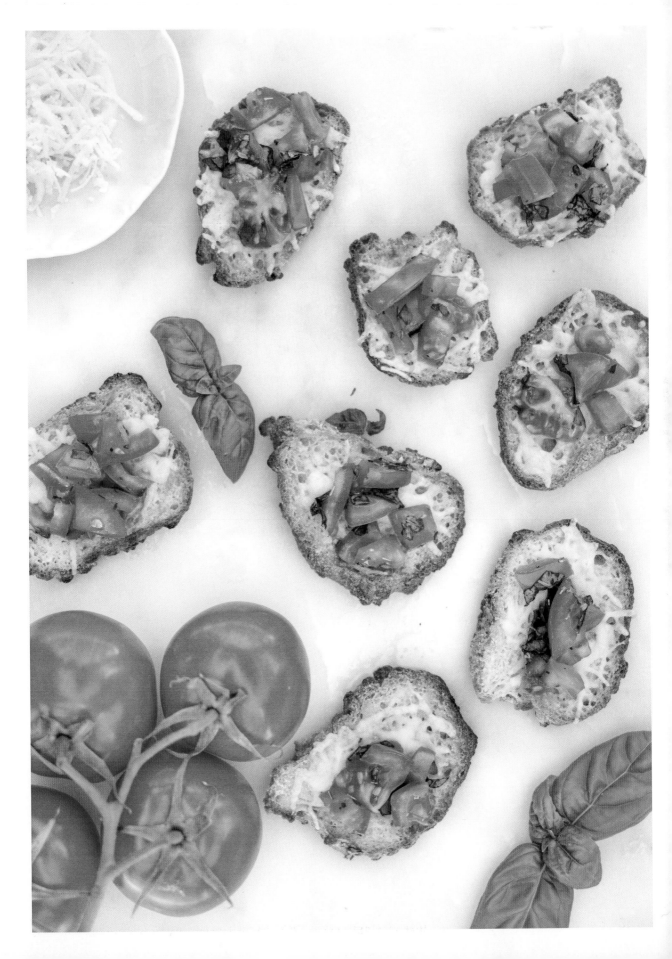

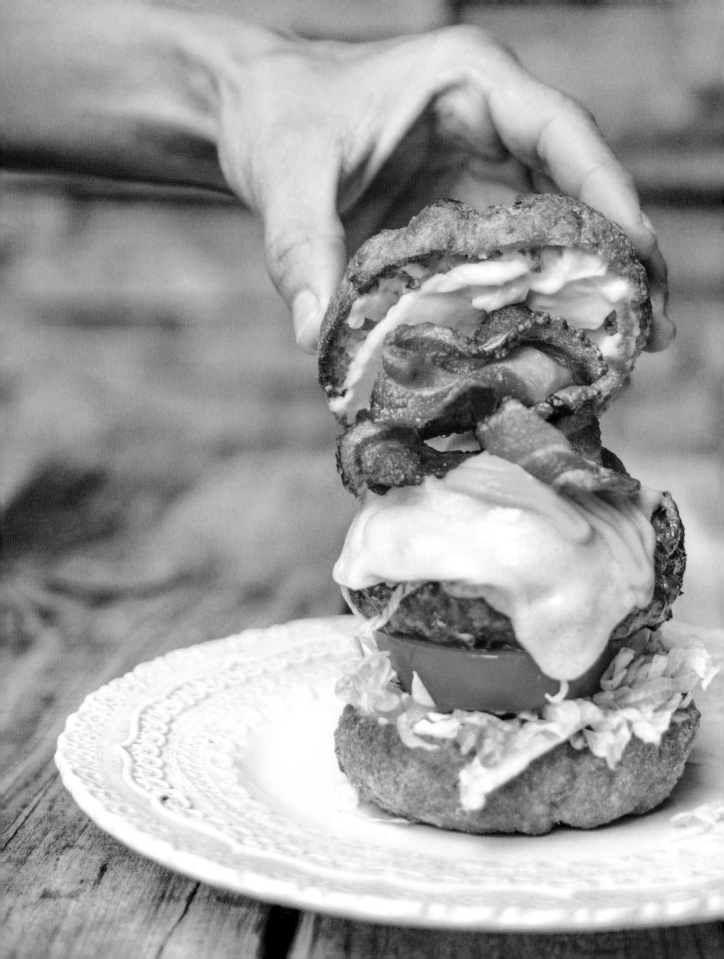

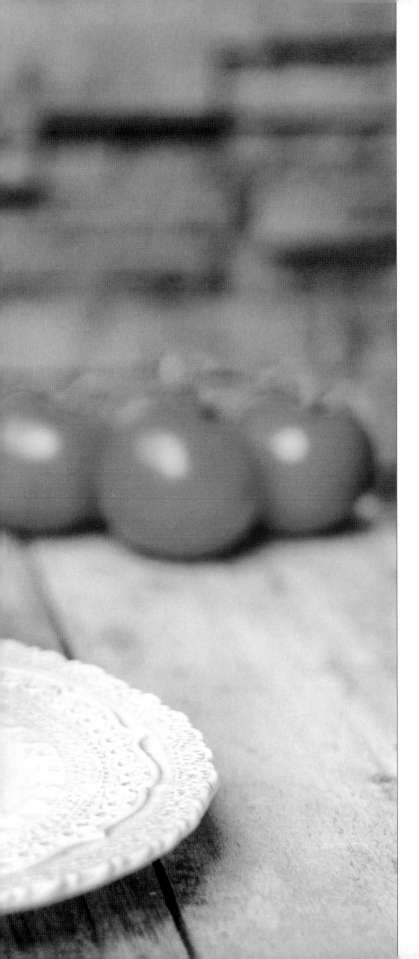

Beef and Lamb

Savory Beefy Poppers

yield: 8 poppers (2 per serving)   *prep time:* 15 minutes   *cook time:* 15 minutes

option   KETO

8 medium jalapeño peppers, stemmed, halved, and seeded

1 (8-ounce) package cream cheese (or Kite Hill brand cream cheese style spread for dairy-free), softened

2 pounds ground beef (85% lean)

1 teaspoon fine sea salt

½ teaspoon ground black pepper

8 slices thin-cut bacon

Fresh cilantro leaves, for garnish

1. Spray the air fryer basket with avocado oil. Preheat the air fryer to 400°F.

2. Stuff each jalapeño half with a few tablespoons of cream cheese. Place the halves back together again to form 8 jalapeños.

3. Season the ground beef with the salt and pepper and mix with your hands to incorporate. Flatten about ¼ pound of ground beef in the palm of your hand and place a stuffed jalapeño in the center. Fold the beef around the jalapeño, forming an egg shape. Wrap the beef-covered jalapeño with a slice of bacon and secure it with a toothpick.

4. Place the jalapeños in the air fryer basket, leaving space between them (if you're using a smaller air fryer, work in batches if necessary), and cook for 15 minutes, or until the beef is cooked through and the bacon is crispy. Garnish with cilantro before serving.

5. Store leftovers in an airtight container in the fridge for 3 days or in the freezer for up to a month. Reheat in a preheated 350°F air fryer for 4 minutes, or until heated through and the bacon is crispy.

note: This recipe was inspired by a similar dish at Agave Kitchen in Hudson, Wisconsin—the owner, Paul, is a fan of keto. Great idea, Paul!

(per serving)   calories **679** | fat **53g** | protein **42g** | total carbs **3g** | fiber **1g**

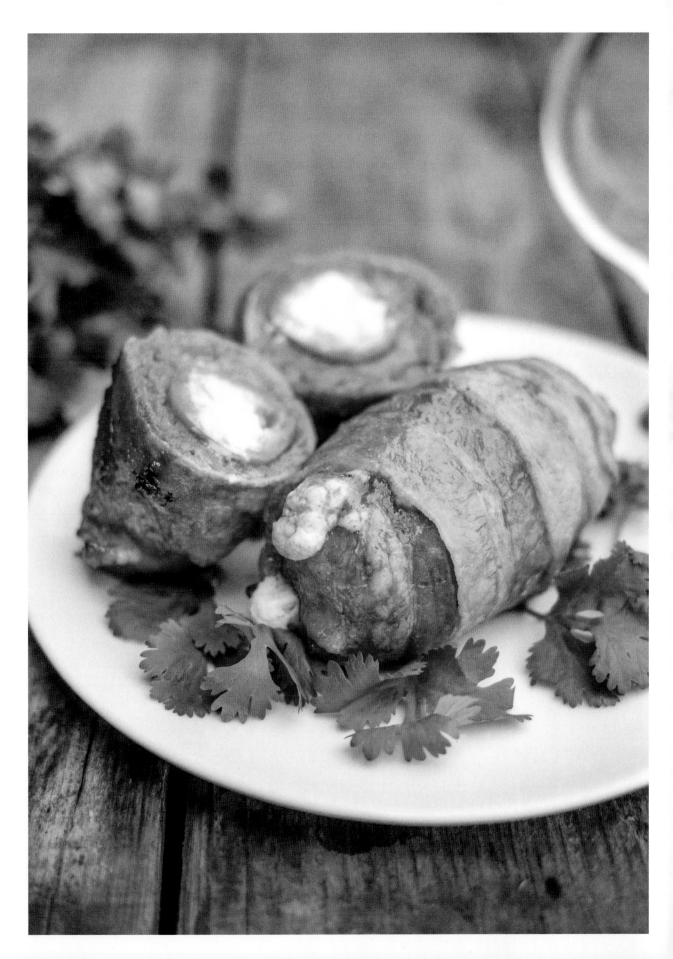

Swedish Meatloaf

yield: 8 servings *prep time:* 10 minutes *cook time:* 35 minutes

option   KETO

1½ pounds ground beef (85% lean)

¼ pound ground pork or ground beef

1 large egg (omit for egg-free)

½ cup minced onions

¼ cup tomato sauce

2 tablespoons dry mustard

2 cloves garlic, minced

2 teaspoons fine sea salt

1 teaspoon ground black pepper, plus more for garnish

SAUCE:

½ cup (1 stick) unsalted butter

½ cup shredded Swiss or mild cheddar cheese (about 2 ounces)

2 ounces cream cheese (¼ cup), softened

⅓ cup beef broth

⅛ teaspoon ground nutmeg

Halved cherry tomatoes, for serving (optional)

1. Preheat the air fryer to 390°F.

2. In a large bowl, combine the ground beef, ground pork, egg, onions, tomato sauce, dry mustard, garlic, salt, and pepper. Using your hands, mix until well combined.

3. Place the meatloaf mixture in a 9 by 5-inch loaf pan and place it in the air fryer. Cook for 35 minutes, or until cooked through and the internal temperature reaches 145°F. Check the meatloaf after 25 minutes; if it's getting too brown on the top, cover it loosely with foil to prevent burning.

4. While the meatloaf cooks, make the sauce: Heat the butter in a saucepan over medium-high heat until it sizzles and brown flecks appear, stirring constantly to keep the butter from burning. Turn the heat down to low and whisk in the Swiss cheese, cream cheese, broth, and nutmeg. Simmer for at least 10 minutes. The longer it simmers, the more the flavors open up.

5. When the meatloaf is done, transfer it to a serving tray and pour the sauce over it. Garnish with ground black pepper and serve with cherry tomatoes, if desired. Allow the meatloaf to rest for 10 minutes before slicing so it doesn't crumble apart.

6. Store leftovers in an airtight container in the fridge for 3 days or in the freezer for up to a month. Reheat in a preheated 350°F air fryer for 4 minutes, or until heated through.

(per serving)   calories **395** | fat **32g** | protein **23g** | total carbs **3g** | fiber **1g**

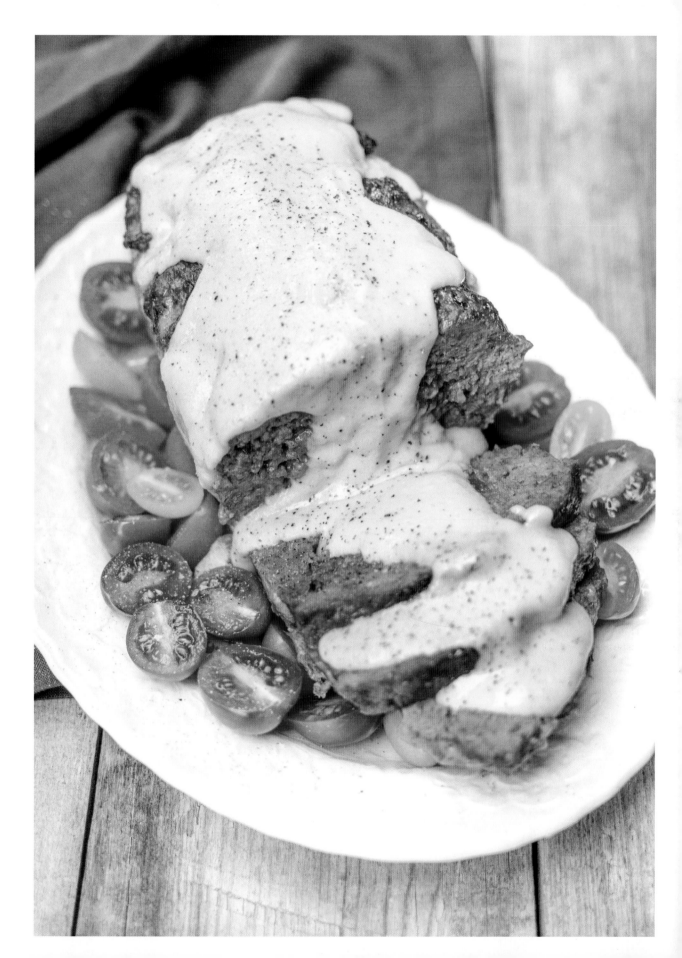

Carne Asada

yield: 4 servings *prep time:* 5 minutes, plus 2 hours to marinate *cook time:* 8 minutes

MARINADE:

1 cup fresh cilantro leaves and stems, plus more for garnish if desired

1 jalapeño pepper, seeded and diced

½ cup lime juice

2 tablespoons avocado oil

2 tablespoons coconut vinegar or apple cider vinegar

2 teaspoons orange extract

1 teaspoon stevia glycerite, or ⅛ teaspoon liquid stevia

2 teaspoons ancho chili powder

2 teaspoons fine sea salt

1 teaspoon coriander seeds

1 teaspoon cumin seeds

1 pound skirt steak, cut into 4 equal portions

FOR SERVING (OPTIONAL):

Chopped avocado

Lime slices

Sliced radishes

1. Make the marinade: Place all the ingredients for the marinade in a blender and puree until smooth.

2. Place the steak in a shallow dish and pour the marinade over it, making sure the meat is covered completely. Cover and place in the fridge for 2 hours or overnight.

3. Spray the air fryer basket with avocado oil. Preheat the air fryer to 400°F.

4. Remove the steak from the marinade and place it in the air fryer basket in one layer. Cook for 8 minutes, or until the internal temperature is 145°F; do not overcook or it will become tough.

5. Remove the steak from the air fryer and place it on a cutting board to rest for 10 minutes before slicing it against the grain. Garnish with cilantro, if desired, and serve with chopped avocado, lime slices, and/or sliced radishes, if desired.

6. Store leftovers in an airtight container in the fridge for 3 days or in the freezer for up to a month. Reheat in a preheated 350°F air fryer for 4 minutes, or until heated through.

(per serving) calories **263** | fat **17g** | protein **24g** | total carbs **4g** | fiber **1g**

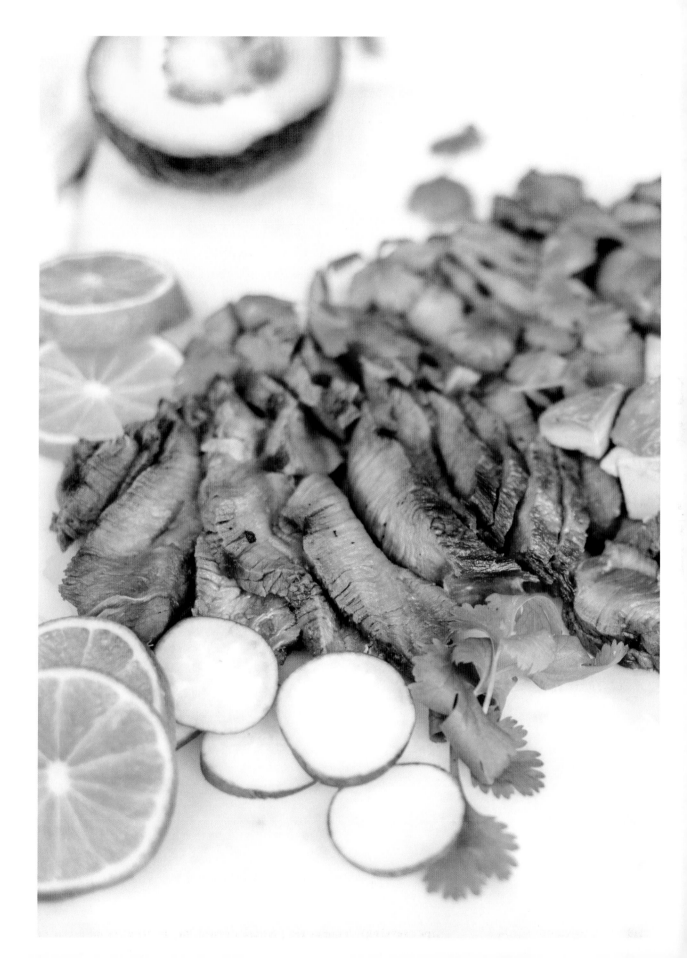

Salisbury Steak with Mushroom Onion Gravy

yield: 2 servings   *prep time:* 10 minutes   *cook time:* 33 minutes
option   KETO

MUSHROOM ONION GRAVY:

¾ cup sliced button mushrooms

¼ cup thinly sliced onions

¼ cup unsalted butter, melted (or bacon fat for dairy-free)

½ teaspoon fine sea salt

¼ cup beef broth

STEAKS:

½ pound ground beef (85% lean)

¼ cup minced onions, or ½ teaspoon onion powder

2 tablespoons tomato paste

1 tablespoon dry mustard

1 clove garlic, minced, or ¼ teaspoon garlic powder

½ teaspoon fine sea salt

¼ teaspoon ground black pepper, plus more for garnish if desired

Chopped fresh thyme leaves, for garnish (optional)

1. Preheat the air fryer to 390°F.

2. Make the gravy: Place the mushrooms and onions in a casserole dish that will fit in your air fryer. Pour the melted butter over them and stir to coat, then season with the salt. Place the dish in the air fryer and cook for 5 minutes, stir, then cook for another 3 minutes, or until the onions are soft and the mushrooms are browning. Add the broth and cook for another 10 minutes.

3. While the gravy is cooking, prepare the steaks: In a large bowl, mix together the ground beef, onions, tomato paste, dry mustard, garlic, salt, and pepper until well combined. Form the mixture into 2 oval-shaped patties.

4. Place the patties on top of the mushroom gravy. Cook for 10 minutes, gently flip the patties, then cook for another 2 to 5 minutes, until the beef is cooked through and the internal temperature reaches 145°F.

5. Transfer the steaks to a serving platter and pour the gravy over them. Garnish with ground black pepper and chopped fresh thyme, if desired. Store leftovers in an airtight container in the fridge for 3 days or in the freezer for up to a month. Reheat in a preheated 350°F air fryer for 4 minutes, or until heated through.

tip: If you have a larger air fryer, you can easily double this recipe to serve four.

(per serving)   calories **588** | fat **44g** | protein **33g** | total carbs **11g** | fiber **3g**

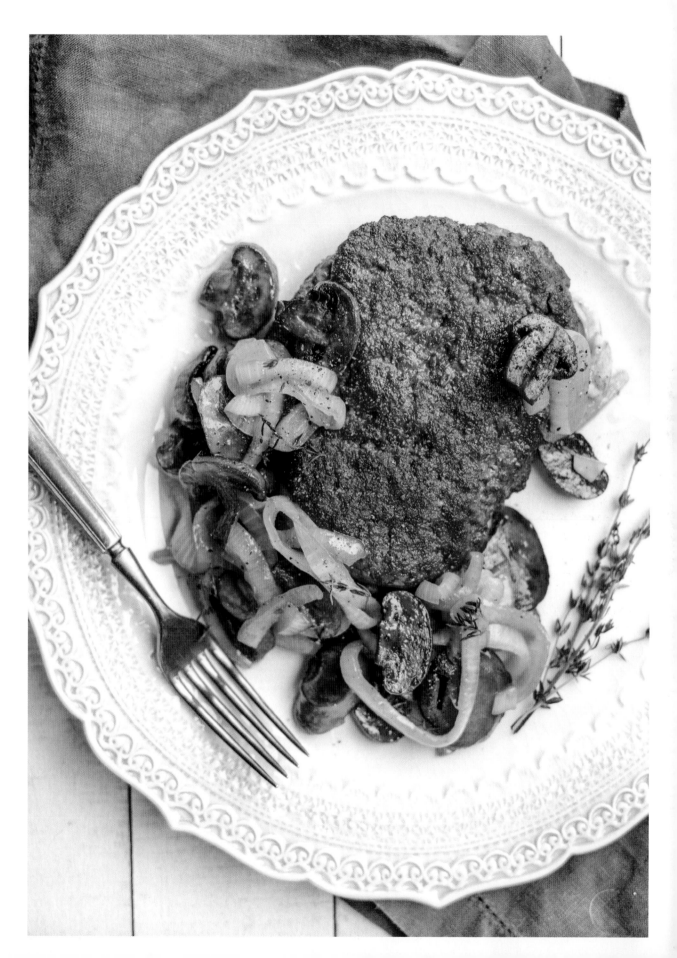

Fajita Meatball Lettuce Wraps

1 pound ground beef (85% lean)

½ cup salsa, plus more for serving if desired

¼ cup chopped onions

¼ cup diced green or red bell peppers

1 large egg, beaten

1 teaspoon fine sea salt

½ teaspoon chili powder

½ teaspoon ground cumin

1 clove garlic, minced

FOR SERVING (OPTIONAL):

8 leaves Boston lettuce

Pico de gallo or salsa

Lime slices

1. Spray the air fryer basket with avocado oil. Preheat the air fryer to 350°F.

2. In a large bowl, mix together all the ingredients until well combined.

3. Shape the meat mixture into eight 1-inch balls. Place the meatballs in the air fryer basket, leaving a little space between them. Cook for 10 minutes, or until cooked through and no longer pink inside and the internal temperature reaches 145°F.

4. Serve each meatball on a lettuce leaf, topped with pico de gallo or salsa, if desired. Serve with lime slices if desired.

5. Store leftovers in an airtight container in the fridge for 3 days or in the freezer for up to a month. Reheat in a preheated 350°F air fryer for 4 minutes, or until heated through.

note: This recipe would also be great as a sub—you can use the recipe for Hot Dog Buns on page 226 for the bread.

(per serving)   calories **272** | fat **18g** | protein **23g** | total carbs **3g** | fiber **0.5g**

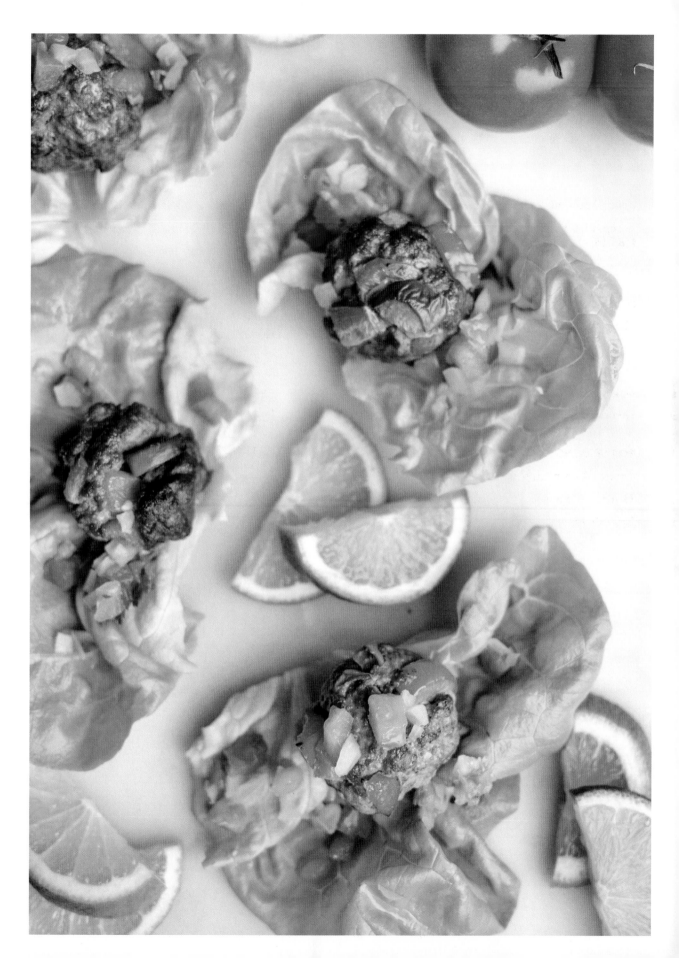

Reuben Fritters

yield: 1 dozen fritters (2 per serving) *prep time:* 10 minutes *cook time:* 16 minutes

2 cups finely diced cooked corned beef

1 (8-ounce) package cream cheese, softened

½ cup finely shredded Swiss cheese (about 2 ounces)

¼ cup sauerkraut

1 cup pork dust (see page 19) or powdered Parmesan cheese (see page 19)

Chopped fresh thyme, for garnish

Thousand Island Dipping Sauce (page 72), for serving (optional; omit for egg-free)

Cornichons, for serving (optional)

1. Spray the air fryer basket with avocado oil. Preheat the air fryer to 390°F.

2. In a large bowl, mix together the corned beef, cream cheese, Swiss cheese, and sauerkraut until well combined. Form the corned beef mixture into twelve 1½-inch balls.

3. Place the pork dust in a shallow bowl. Roll the corned beef balls in the pork dust and use your hands to form it into a thick crust around each ball.

4. Place 6 balls in the air fryer basket, spaced about ½ inch apart, and cook for 8 minutes, or until golden brown and crispy. Allow them to cool a bit before lifting them out of the air fryer (the fritters are very soft when the cheese is melted; they're easier to handle once the cheese has hardened a bit). Repeat with the remaining fritters.

5. Garnish with chopped fresh thyme and serve with the dipping sauce and cornichons, if desired. Store leftovers in an airtight container in the fridge for 3 days or in the freezer for up to a month. Reheat in a preheated 350°F air fryer for 4 minutes, or until heated through.

tip: To make it even easier to form the fritters, refrigerate the corned beef mixture for at least 2 hours or overnight.

(per serving)   calories **527** | fat **50g** | protein **18g** | total carbs **2g** | fiber **0.1g**

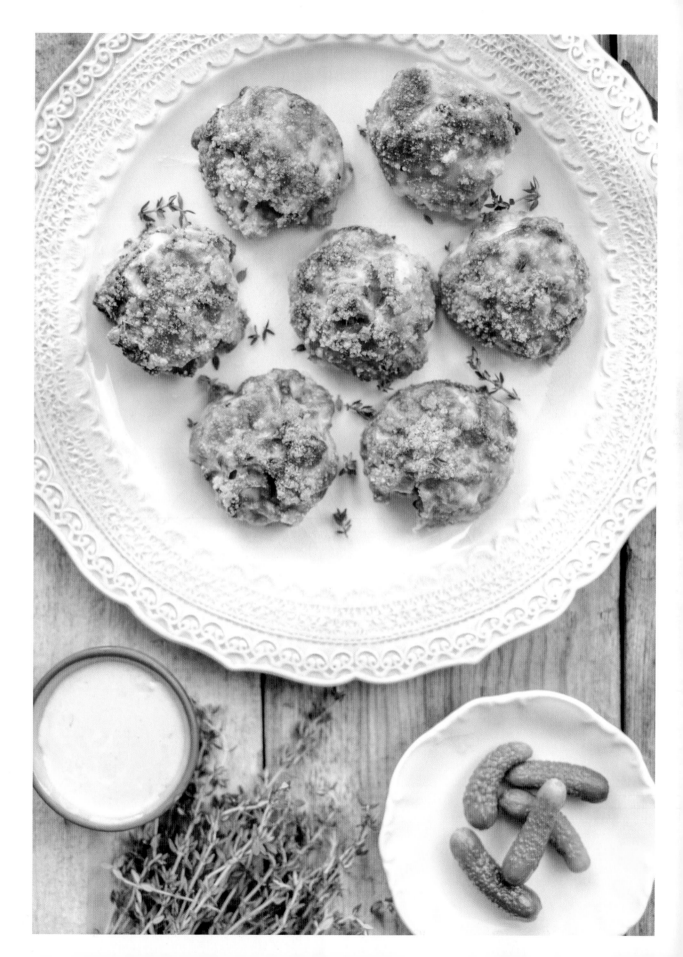

Greek Stuffed Tenderloin

yield: 4 servings *prep time:* 10 minutes *cook time:* 10 minutes

1½ pounds venison or beef tenderloin, pounded to ¼ inch thick

3 teaspoons fine sea salt

1 teaspoon ground black pepper

2 ounces creamy goat cheese

½ cup crumbled feta cheese (about 2 ounces)

¼ cup finely chopped onions

2 cloves garlic, minced

FOR GARNISH/SERVING (OPTIONAL):

Prepared yellow mustard

Halved cherry tomatoes

Extra-virgin olive oil

Sprigs of fresh rosemary

Lavender flowers

1. Spray the air fryer basket with avocado oil. Preheat the air fryer to 400°F.

2. Season the tenderloin on all sides with the salt and pepper.

3. In a medium-sized mixing bowl, combine the goat cheese, feta, onions, and garlic. Place the mixture in the center of the tenderloin. Starting at the end closest to you, tightly roll the tenderloin like a jelly roll. Tie the rolled tenderloin tightly with kitchen twine.

4. Place the meat in the air fryer basket and cook for 5 minutes. Flip the meat over and cook for another 5 minutes, or until the internal temperature reaches 135°F for medium-rare.

5. To serve, smear a line of prepared yellow mustard on a platter, then place the meat next to it and add halved cherry tomatoes on the side, if desired. Drizzle with olive oil and garnish with rosemary sprigs and lavender flowers, if desired.

6. Best served fresh. Store leftovers in an airtight container in the fridge for 3 days. Reheat in a preheated 350°F air fryer for 4 minutes, or until heated through.

(per serving)   calories **415** | fat **16g** | protein **62g** | total carbs **4g** | fiber **0.3g**

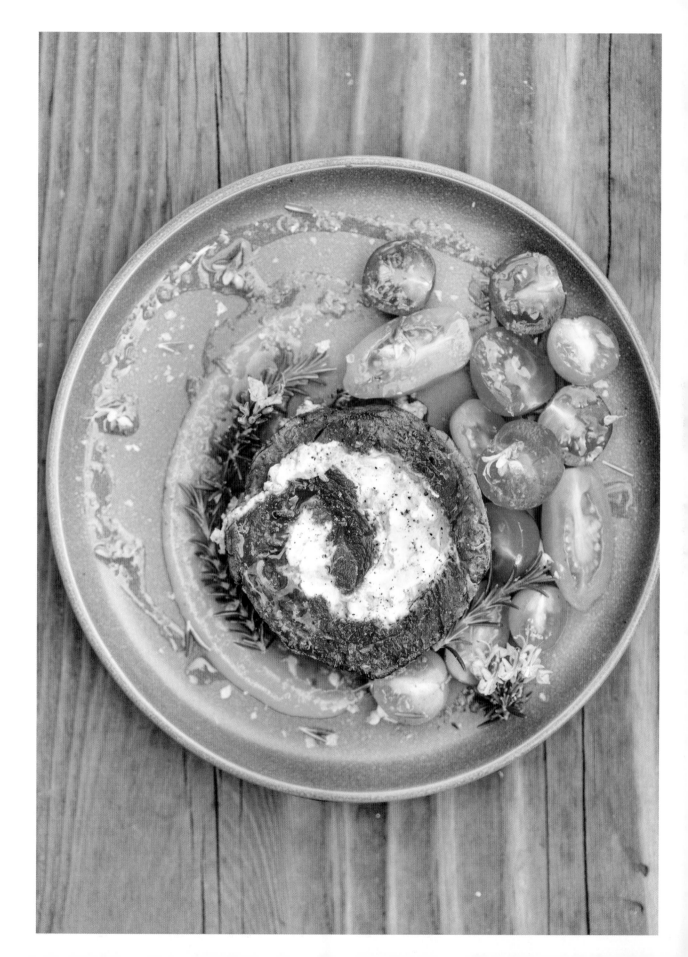

Herb-Crusted Lamb Chops

yield: 2 servings *prep time:* 10 minutes *cook time:* 5 minutes

1 large egg

2 cloves garlic, minced

¼ cup pork dust (see page 19)

¼ cup powdered Parmesan cheese (see page 19) (or pork dust for dairy-free; see page 19)

1 tablespoon chopped fresh oregano leaves

1 tablespoon chopped fresh rosemary leaves

1 teaspoon chopped fresh thyme leaves

½ teaspoon ground black pepper

4 (1-inch-thick) lamb chops

FOR GARNISH/SERVING (OPTIONAL):

Sprigs of fresh oregano

Sprigs of fresh rosemary

Sprigs of fresh thyme

Lavender flowers

Lemon slices

1. Spray the air fryer basket with avocado oil. Preheat the air fryer to 400°F.

2. Beat the egg in a shallow bowl, add the garlic, and stir well to combine. In another shallow bowl, mix together the pork dust, Parmesan, herbs, and pepper.

3. One at a time, dip the lamb chops into the egg mixture, shake off the excess egg, and then dredge them in the Parmesan mixture. Use your hands to coat the chops well in the Parmesan mixture and form a nice crust on all sides; if necessary, dip the chops again in both the egg and the Parmesan mixture.

4. Place the lamb chops in the air fryer basket, leaving space between them, and cook for 5 minutes, or until the internal temperature reaches 145°F for medium doneness. Allow to rest for 10 minutes before serving.

5. Garnish with sprigs of oregano, rosemary, and thyme, and lavender flowers, if desired. Serve with lemon slices, if desired.

6. Best served fresh. Store leftovers in an airtight container in the fridge for up to 4 days. Serve chilled over a salad, or reheat in a 350°F air fryer for 3 minutes, or until heated through.

(per serving)   calories **790** | fat **60g** | protein **57g** | total carbs **2g** | fiber **0.4g**

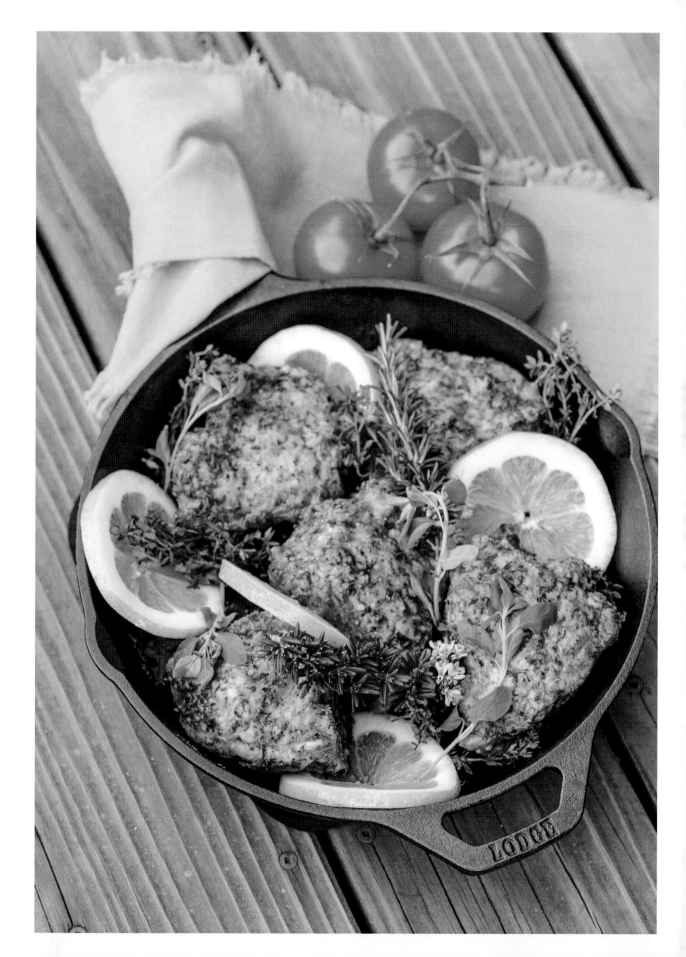

Black 'n' Blue Burgers

option KETO

yield: 2 servings *prep time:* 5 minutes *cook time:* 10 minutes

½ teaspoon fine sea salt

¼ teaspoon ground black pepper

¼ teaspoon garlic powder

¼ teaspoon onion powder

¼ teaspoon smoked paprika

2 (¼-pound) hamburger patties, ½ inch thick

½ cup crumbled blue cheese (about 2 ounces) (omit for dairy-free)

2 Hamburger Buns (page 226)

2 tablespoons mayonnaise

6 red onion slices

2 Boston lettuce leaves

1. Spray the air fryer basket with avocado oil. Preheat the air fryer to 360°F.

2. In a small bowl, combine the salt, pepper, and seasonings. Season the patties well on both sides with the seasoning mixture.

3. Place the patties in the air fryer basket and cook for 7 minutes, or until the internal temperature reaches 145°F for a medium-done burger. Place the blue cheese on top of the patties and cook for another minute to melt the cheese. Remove the burgers from the air fryer and allow to rest for 5 minutes.

4. Slice the buns in half and smear 2 halves with a tablespoon of mayo each. Increase the heat to 400°F and place the buns in the air fryer basket cut side up. Toast the buns for 1 to 2 minutes, until golden brown.

5. Remove the buns from the air fryer and place them on a serving plate. Place the burgers on the buns and top each burger with 3 red onion slices and a lettuce leaf.

6. Best served fresh. Store leftover patties in an airtight container in the fridge for 3 days or in the freezer for up to a month. Reheat in a preheated 350°F air fryer for 4 minutes, or until heated through.

(per serving) calories **237** | fat **20g** | protein **11g** | total carbs **3g** | fiber **1g**

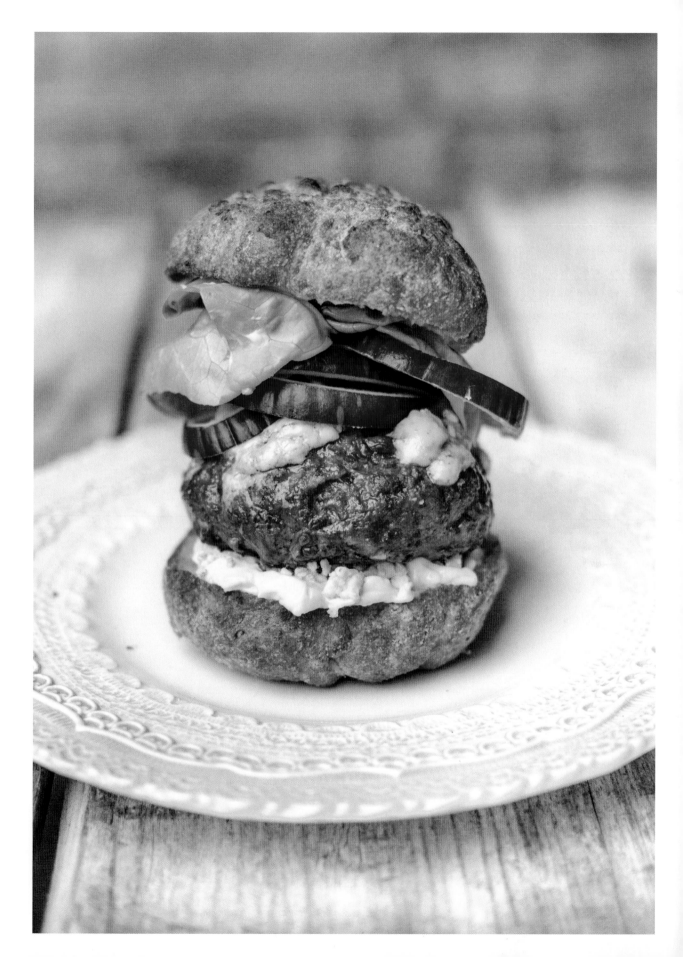

Mojito Lamb Chops

MARINADE:

2 teaspoons grated lime zest

½ cup lime juice

¼ cup avocado oil

¼ cup chopped fresh mint leaves

4 cloves garlic, roughly chopped

2 teaspoons fine sea salt

½ teaspoon ground black pepper

4 (1-inch-thick) lamb chops

Sprigs of fresh mint, for garnish (optional)

Lime slices, for serving (optional)

1. Make the marinade: Place all the ingredients for the marinade in a food processor or blender and puree until mostly smooth with a few small chunks. Transfer half of the marinade to a shallow dish and set the other half aside for serving. Add the lamb to the shallow dish, cover, and place in the refrigerator to marinate for at least 2 hours or overnight.

2. Spray the air fryer basket with avocado oil. Preheat the air fryer to 390°F.

3. Remove the chops from the marinade and place them in the air fryer basket. Cook for 5 minutes, or until the internal temperature reaches 145°F for medium doneness.

4. Allow the chops to rest for 10 minutes before serving with the rest of the marinade as a sauce. Garnish with fresh mint leaves and serve with lime slices, if desired. Best served fresh.

(per serving) calories **692** | fat **53g** | protein **48g** | total carbs **2g** | fiber **0.4g**

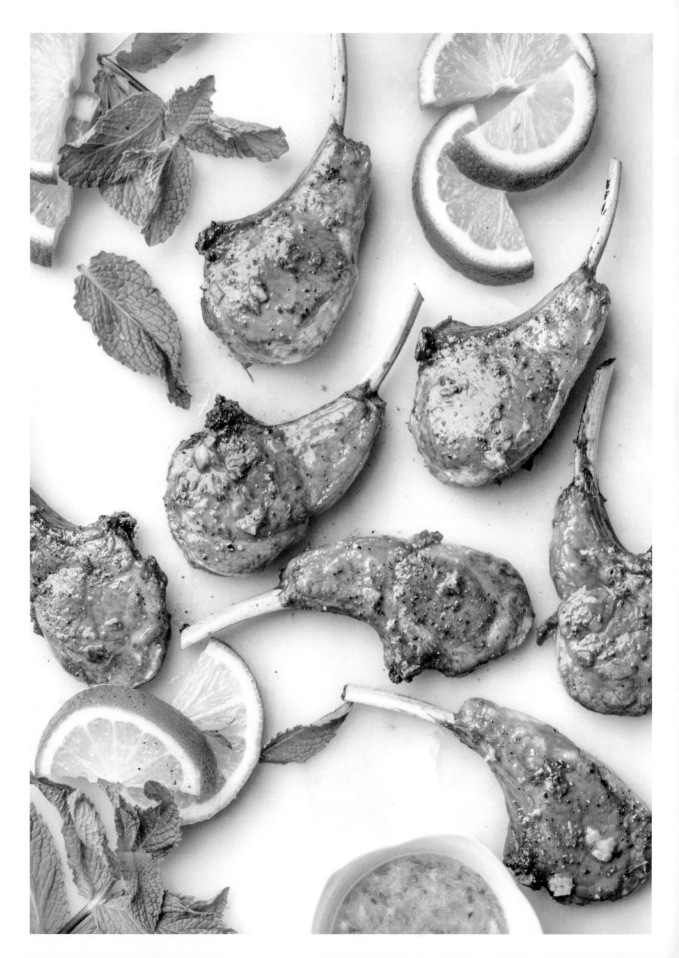

Mushroom and Swiss Burgers

yield: 2 servings   *prep time:* 5 minutes   *cook time:* 15 minutes

2 large portobello mushrooms

1 teaspoon fine sea salt, divided

¼ teaspoon garlic powder

¼ teaspoon ground black pepper

¼ teaspoon onion powder

¼ teaspoon smoked paprika

2 (¼-pound) hamburger patties, ½ inch thick

2 slices Swiss cheese (omit for dairy-free)

Condiments of choice, such as Ranch Dressing (page 68; use dairy-free if needed), prepared yellow mustard, or mayonnaise, for serving

1. Preheat the air fryer to 360°F.

2. Clean the portobello mushrooms and remove the stems. Spray the mushrooms on all sides with avocado oil and season them with ½ teaspoon of the salt. Place the mushrooms in the air fryer basket and cook for 7 to 8 minutes, until fork-tender and soft to the touch.

3. While the mushrooms cook, in a small bowl mix together the remaining ½ teaspoon of salt, the garlic powder, pepper, onion powder, and paprika. Sprinkle the hamburger patties with the seasoning mixture.

4. When the mushrooms are done cooking, remove them from the air fryer and place them on a serving platter with the cap side down.

5. Place the hamburger patties in the air fryer and cook for 7 minutes, or until the internal temperature reaches 145°F for a medium-done burger. Place a slice of Swiss cheese on each patty and cook for another minute to melt the cheese.

6. Place the burgers on top of the mushrooms and drizzle with condiments of your choice. Best served fresh.

(per serving)   calories **345** | fat **23g** | protein **30g** | total carbs **5g** | fiber **1g**

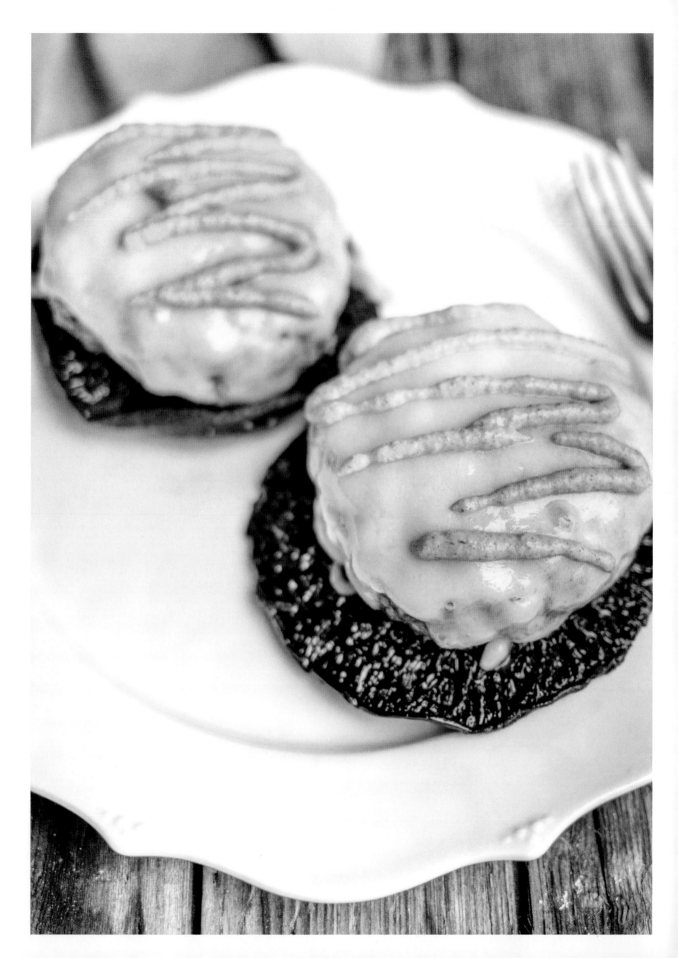

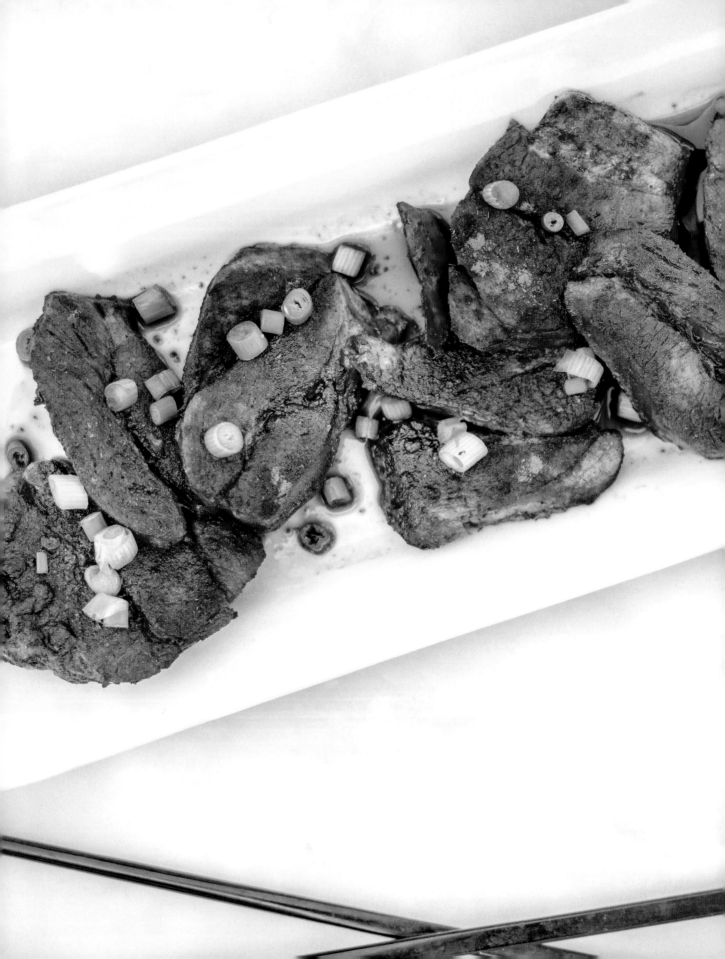

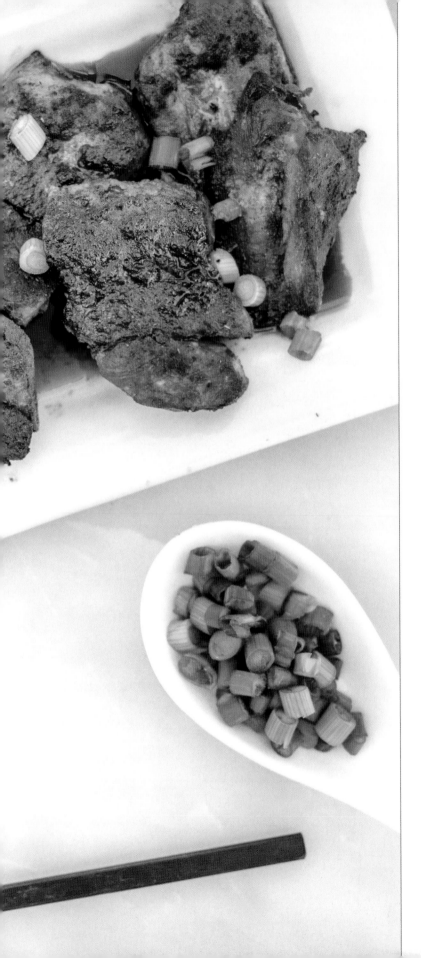

Pork

Deconstructed Chicago Dogs

yield: 4 servings   *prep time:* 10 minutes   *cook time:* 7 minutes

4 hot dogs

2 large dill pickles

¼ cup diced onions

1 tomato, cut into ½-inch dice

4 pickled sport peppers, diced

FOR GARNISH (OPTIONAL):

Brown mustard

Celery salt

Poppy seeds

1. Spray the air fryer basket with avocado oil. Preheat the air fryer to 400°F.

2. Place the hot dogs in the air fryer basket and cook for 5 to 7 minutes, until hot and slightly crispy.

3. While the hot dogs cook, quarter one of the dill pickles lengthwise, so that you have 4 pickle spears. Finely dice the other pickle.

4. When the hot dogs are done, transfer them to a serving platter and arrange them in a row, alternating with the pickle spears. Top with the diced pickles, onions, tomato, and sport peppers. Drizzle brown mustard on top and garnish with celery salt and poppy seeds, if desired.

5. Best served fresh. Store leftover hot dogs in an airtight container in the refrigerator for up to 3 days. Reheat in a preheated 390°F air fryer for 2 minutes, or until warmed through.

(per serving)   calories **123** | fat **8g** | protein **8g** | total carbs **3g** | fiber **1g**

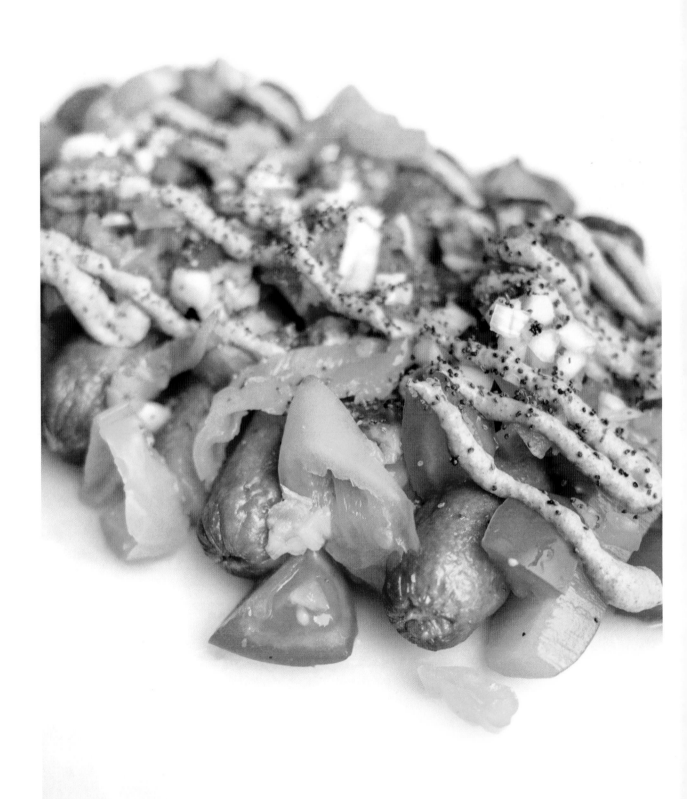

Pork Milanese

yield: 4 servings *prep time:* 10 minutes *cook time:* 12 minutes

option   KETO

4 (1-inch) boneless pork chops

Fine sea salt and ground black pepper

2 large eggs

¾ cup powdered Parmesan cheese (about 2¼ ounces; see page 19) (or pork dust for dairy-free; see page 19)

Chopped fresh parsley, for garnish

Lemon slices, for serving

1. Spray the air fryer basket with avocado oil. Preheat the air fryer to 400°F.

2. Place the pork chops between 2 sheets of plastic wrap and pound them with the flat side of a meat tenderizer until they're ¼ inch thick. Lightly season both sides of the chops with salt and pepper.

3. Lightly beat the eggs in a shallow bowl. Divide the Parmesan cheese evenly between 2 bowls and set the bowls in this order: Parmesan, eggs, Parmesan. Dredge a chop in the first bowl of Parmesan, then dip it in the eggs, and then dredge it again in the second bowl of Parmesan, making sure both sides and all edges are well coated. Repeat with the remaining chops.

4. Place the chops in the air fryer basket and cook for 12 minutes, or until the internal temperature reaches 145°F, flipping halfway through.

5. Garnish with fresh parsley and serve immediately with lemon slices. Store leftovers in an airtight container in the refrigerator for up to 3 days. Reheat in a preheated 390°F air fryer for 5 minutes, or until warmed through.

tip: Ask your butcher to pound the chops thin for you. Then all you have to do is dip them in the breading and fry them for a tasty dinner.

(per serving) calories 351 | fat 18g | protein 42g | total carbs 3g | fiber 1g

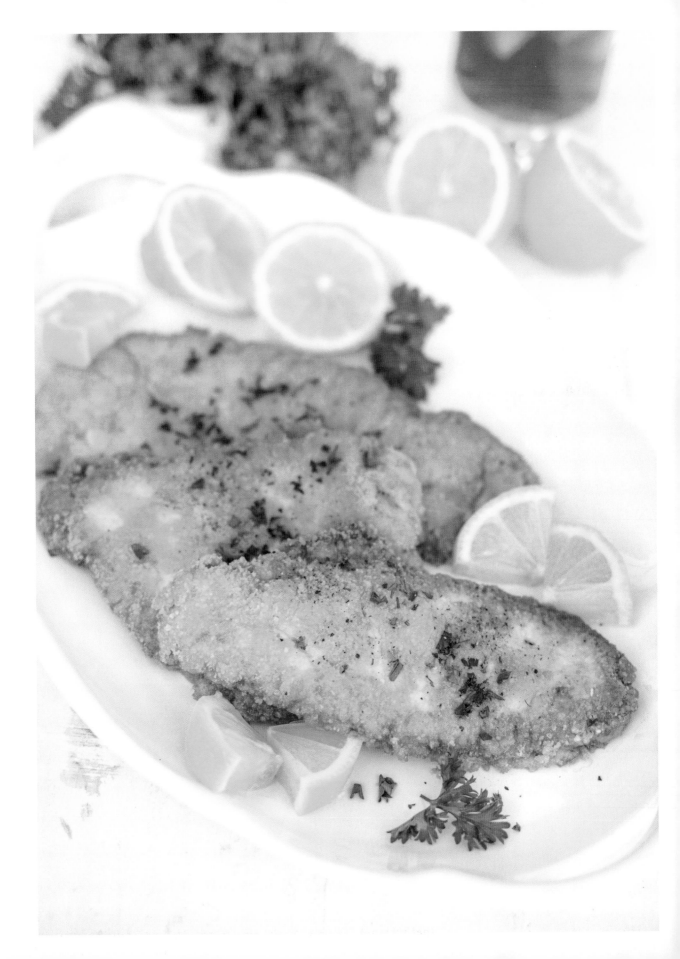

Italian Sausages with Peppers and Onions

yield: 3 servings   *prep time:* 5 minutes   *cook time:* 28 minutes

1 medium onion, thinly sliced

1 yellow or orange bell pepper, thinly sliced

1 red bell pepper, thinly sliced

¼ cup avocado oil or melted coconut oil

1 teaspoon fine sea salt

6 Italian sausages

Dijon mustard, for serving (optional)

1. Preheat the air fryer to 400°F.

2. Place the onion and peppers in a large bowl. Drizzle with the oil and toss well to coat the veggies. Season with the salt.

3. Place the onion and peppers in a 6-inch pie pan and cook in the air fryer for 8 minutes, stirring halfway through. Remove from the air fryer and set aside.

4. Spray the air fryer basket with avocado oil. Place the sausages in the air fryer basket and cook for 20 minutes, or until crispy and golden brown. During the last minute or two of cooking, add the onion and peppers to the basket with the sausages to warm them through.

5. Place the onion and peppers on a serving platter and arrange the sausages on top. Serve Dijon mustard on the side, if desired.

6. Store leftovers in an airtight container in the fridge for up to 7 days or in the freezer for up to a month. Reheat in a preheated 390°F air fryer for 3 minutes, or until heated through.

(per serving)   calories **576** | fat **49g** | protein **25g** | total carbs **8g** | fiber **2g**

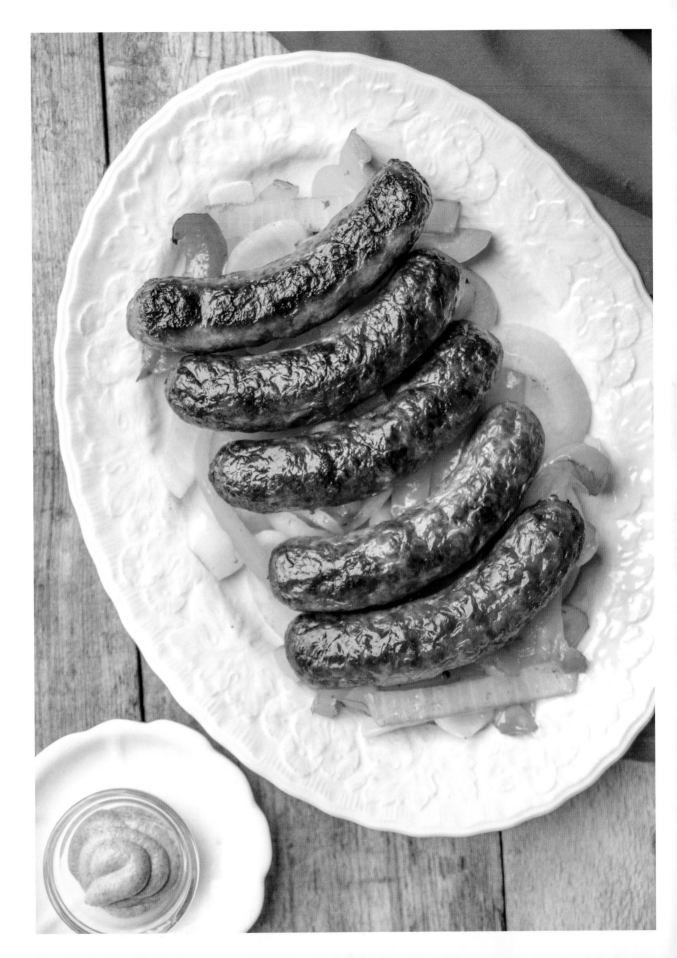

Scotch Eggs

yield: 8 eggs (1 per serving) *prep time:* 10 minutes *cook time:* 15 minutes

2 pounds ground pork or ground beef

2 teaspoons fine sea salt

½ teaspoon ground black pepper, plus more for garnish

8 large hard-boiled eggs, peeled

2 cups pork dust (see page 19)

Dijon mustard, for serving (optional)

1. Spray the air fryer basket with avocado oil. Preheat the air fryer to 400°F.

2. Place the ground pork in a large bowl, add the salt and pepper, and use your hands to mix until seasoned throughout. Flatten about ¼ pound of ground pork in the palm of your hand and place a peeled egg in the center. Fold the pork completely around the egg. Repeat with the remaining eggs.

3. Place the pork dust in a medium-sized bowl. One at a time, roll the ground pork–covered eggs in the pork dust and use your hands to press it into the eggs to form a nice crust. Place the eggs in the air fryer basket and spray them with avocado oil.

4. Cook the eggs for 15 minutes, or until the internal temperature of the pork reaches 145°F and the outside is golden brown. Garnish with ground black pepper and serve with Dijon mustard, if desired.

5. Store leftovers in an airtight container in the fridge for up to 7 days or in the freezer for up to a month. Reheat in a preheated 400°F air fryer for 3 minutes, or until heated through.

(per serving)   calories **447** | fat **34g** | protein **43g** | total carbs **0.5g** | fiber **0g**

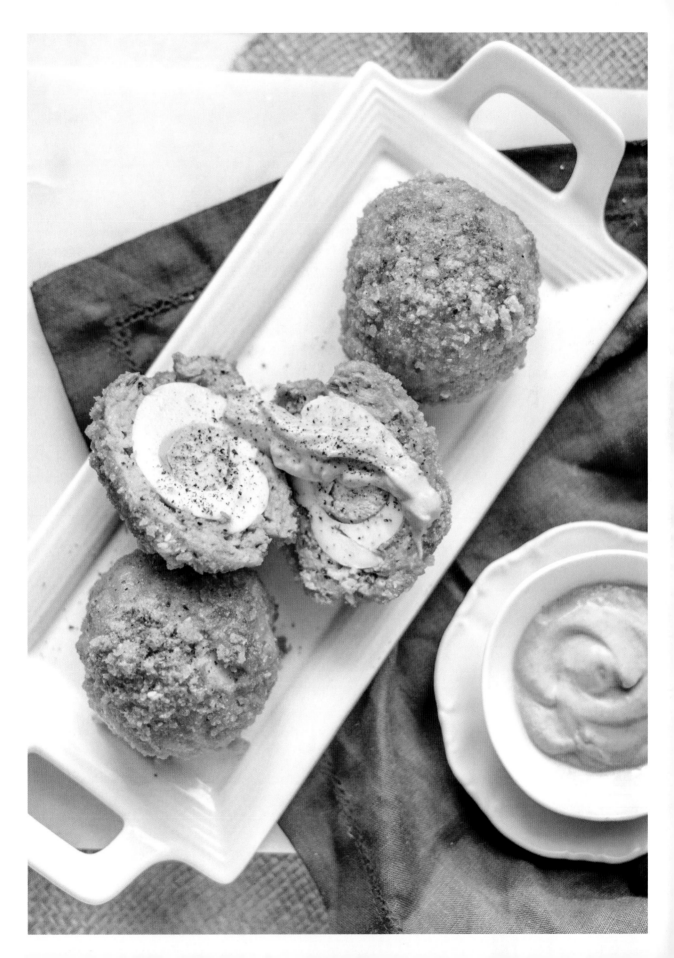

Mama Maria's Savory Sausage Cobbler

yield: 4 servings *prep time:* 15 minutes *cook time:* 34 minutes

KETO

FILLING:

1 pound ground Italian sausage

1 cup sliced mushrooms

1 teaspoon fine sea salt

2 cups marinara sauce

BISCUITS:

3 large egg whites

¾ cup blanched almond flour

1 teaspoon baking powder

¼ teaspoon fine sea salt

2½ tablespoons very cold unsalted butter, cut into ¼-inch pieces (see Tip)

Fresh basil leaves, for garnish

tip: Make sure that the butter for the biscuits is very cold; if it's not, the biscuits won't turn out.

1. Preheat the air fryer to 400°F.

2. Place the sausage in a 7-inch pie pan (or a pan that fits into your air fryer). Use your hands to break up the sausage and spread it evenly on the bottom of the pan. Place the pan in the air fryer and cook for 5 minutes.

3. Remove the pan from the air fryer and use a fork or metal spatula to crumble the sausage more. Season the mushrooms with the salt and add them to the pie pan. Stir to combine the mushrooms and sausage, then return the pan to the air fryer and cook for 4 minutes, or until the mushrooms are soft and the sausage is cooked through.

4. Remove the pan from the air fryer. Add the marinara sauce and stir well. Set aside.

5. Make the biscuits: Place the egg whites in a large mixing bowl or the bowl of a stand mixer. Using a hand mixer or stand mixer, whip the egg whites until stiff peaks form.

6. In a medium-sized bowl, whisk together the almond flour, baking powder, and salt, then cut in the butter. Gently fold the flour mixture into the egg whites with a rubber spatula.

7. Using a large spoon or ice cream scoop, spoon one-quarter of the dough on top of the sausage mixture, making sure the butter stays in separate clumps. Repeat with the remaining dough, spacing the biscuits about 1 inch apart.

8. Place the pan in the air fryer and cook for 5 minutes, then lower the heat to 325°F and cook for another 15 to 20 minutes, until the biscuits are golden brown. Serve garnished with fresh basil leaves.

9. Store leftovers in an airtight container in the refrigerator for up to 3 days. Reheat in a preheated 350°F air fryer for 5 minutes, or until warmed through.

(per serving)   calories **588** | fat **48g** | protein **28g** | total carbs **9g** | fiber **3g**

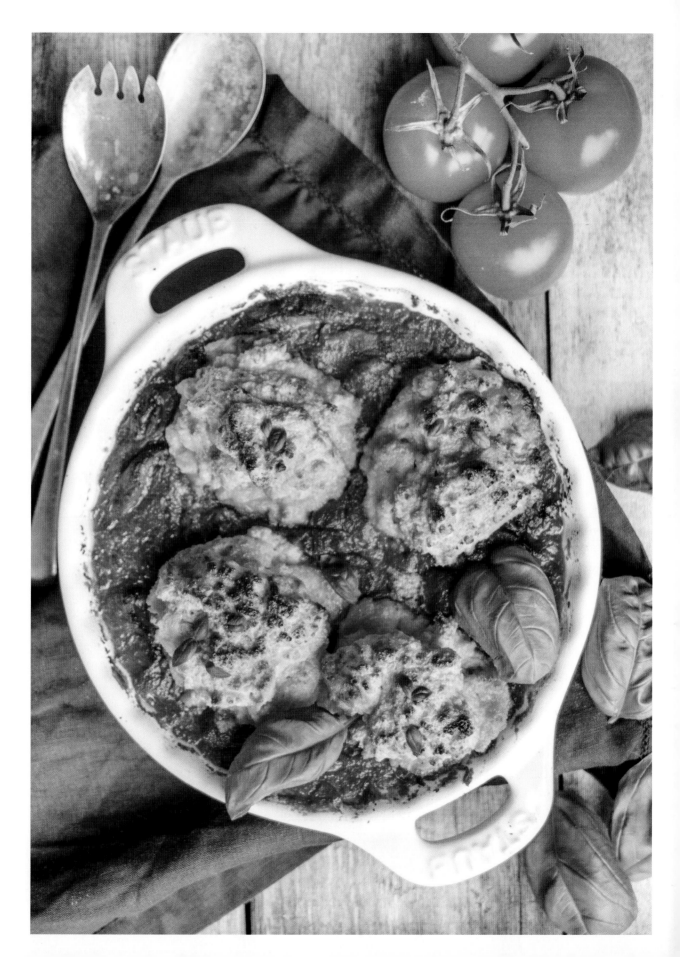

Pork Tenderloin with Avocado Lime Sauce

yield: 4 servings   *prep time:* 10 minutes, plus 2 hours to marinate   *cook time:* 15 minutes

   option   KETO

MARINADE:

½ cup lime juice

Grated zest of 1 lime

2 teaspoons stevia glycerite, or ¼ teaspoon liquid stevia

3 cloves garlic, minced

1½ teaspoons fine sea salt

1 teaspoon chili powder, or more for more heat

1 teaspoon smoked paprika

1 pound pork tenderloin

AVOCADO LIME SAUCE:

1 medium-sized ripe avocado, roughly chopped

½ cup full-fat sour cream (or coconut cream for dairy-free)

Grated zest of 1 lime

Juice of 1 lime

2 cloves garlic, roughly chopped

½ teaspoon fine sea salt

¼ teaspoon ground black pepper

Chopped fresh cilantro leaves, for garnish

Lime slices, for serving

Pico de gallo, for serving

1. In a medium-sized casserole dish, stir together all the marinade ingredients until well combined. Add the tenderloin and coat it well in the marinade. Cover and place in the fridge to marinate for 2 hours or overnight.

2. Spray the air fryer basket with avocado oil. Preheat the air fryer to 400°F.

3. Remove the pork from the marinade and place it in the air fryer basket. Cook for 13 to 15 minutes, until the internal temperature of the pork is 145°F, flipping after 7 minutes. Remove the pork from the air fryer and place it on a cutting board. Allow it to rest for 8 to 10 minutes, then cut it into ½-inch-thick slices.

4. While the pork cooks, make the avocado lime sauce: Place all the sauce ingredients in a food processor and puree until smooth. Taste and adjust the seasoning to your liking.

5. Place the pork slices on a serving platter and spoon the avocado lime sauce on top. Garnish with cilantro leaves and serve with lime slices and pico de gallo.

6. Store leftovers in an airtight container in the fridge for up to 4 days. Reheat in a preheated 400°F air fryer for 5 minutes, or until heated through.

(per serving)   calories **326** | fat **19g** | protein **26g** | total carbs **15g** | fiber **6g**

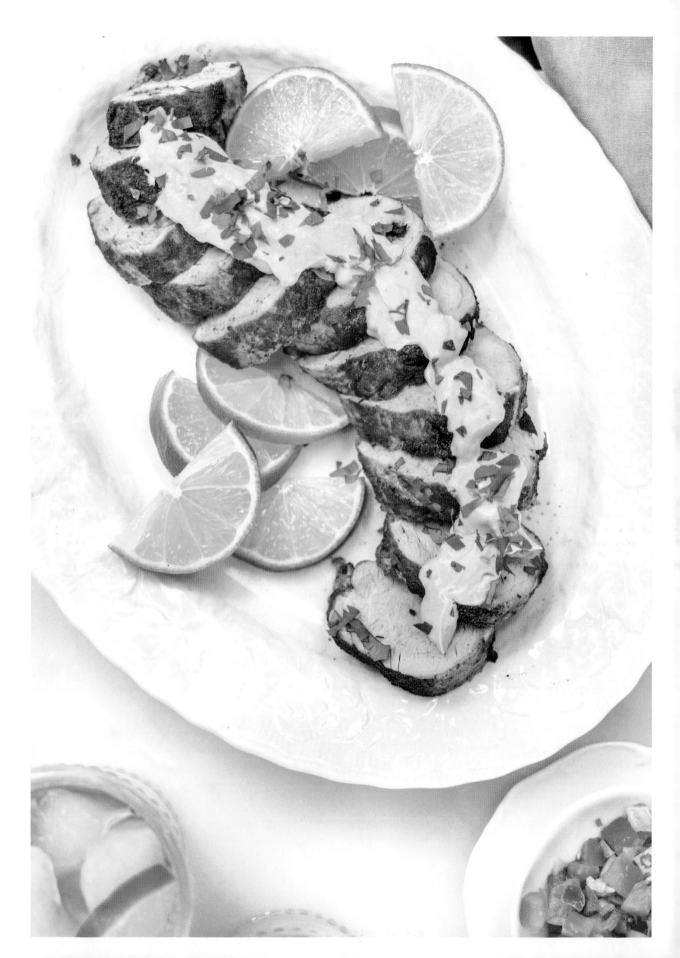

Five-Spice Pork Belly

yield: 4 servings   *prep time:* 10 minutes   *cook time:* 17 minutes

1 pound unsalted pork belly

2 teaspoons Chinese five-spice powder

SAUCE:

1 tablespoon coconut oil

1 (1-inch) piece fresh ginger, peeled and grated

2 cloves garlic, minced

½ cup beef or chicken broth

¼ to ½ cup Swerve confectioners'-style sweetener or equivalent amount of liquid or powdered sweetener (see page 18)

3 tablespoons wheat-free tamari, or ½ cup coconut aminos

1 green onion, sliced, plus more for garnish

1 drop orange oil, or ½ teaspoon orange extract (optional)

1. Spray the air fryer basket with avocado oil. Preheat the air fryer to 400°F.

2. Cut the pork belly into ½-inch-thick slices and season well on all sides with the five-spice powder. Place the slices in a single layer in the air fryer basket (if you're using a smaller air fryer, work in batches if necessary) and cook for 8 minutes, or until cooked to your liking, flipping halfway through.

3. While the pork belly cooks, make the sauce: Heat the coconut oil in a small saucepan over medium heat. Add the ginger and garlic and sauté for 1 minute, or until fragrant. Add the broth, sweetener, and tamari and simmer for 10 to 15 minutes, until thickened. Add the green onion and cook for another minute, until the green onion is softened. Add the orange oil (if using). Taste and adjust the seasoning to your liking.

4. Transfer the pork belly to a large bowl. Pour the sauce over the pork belly and coat well. Place the pork belly slices on a serving platter and garnish with sliced green onions.

5. Best served fresh. Store leftovers in an airtight container in the fridge for up to 4 days. Reheat in a preheated 400°F air fryer for 3 minutes, or until heated through.

(per serving)   calories **365** | fat **32g** | protein **19g** | total carbs **2g** | fiber **0.3g**

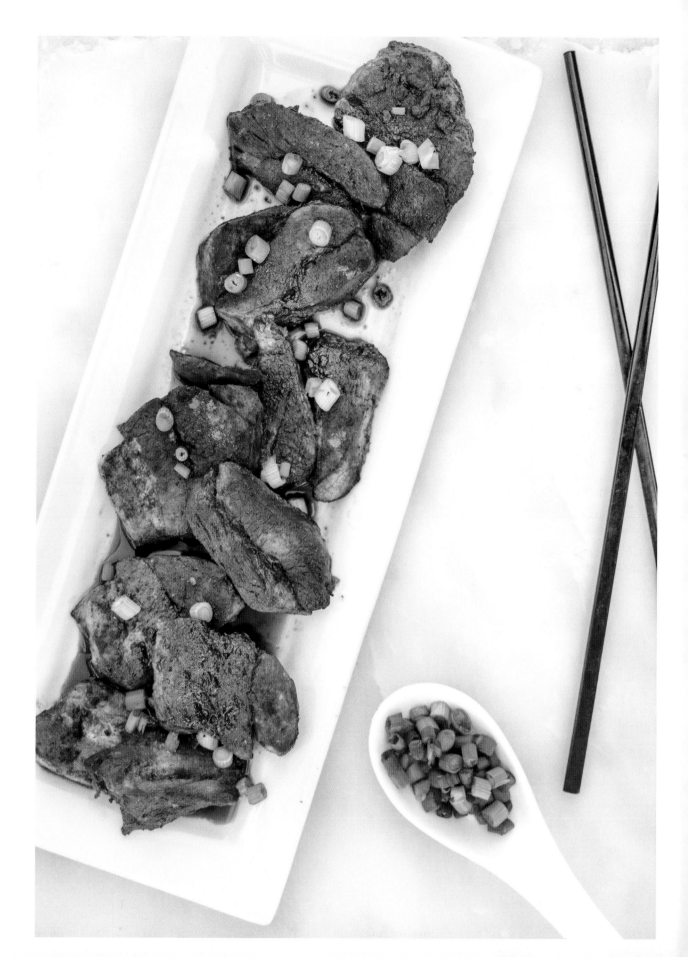

BBQ Riblets

1 rack pork riblets, cut into individual riblets (see Note)

1 teaspoon fine sea salt

1 teaspoon ground black pepper

SAUCE:

¼ cup apple cider vinegar

¼ cup beef broth

¼ cup Swerve confectioners'-style sweetener or equivalent amount of liquid or powdered sweetener (see page 18)

¼ cup tomato sauce

1 teaspoon liquid smoke

1 teaspoon onion powder

2 cloves garlic, minced

1. Spray the air fryer basket with avocado oil. Preheat the air fryer to 350°F.

2. Season the riblets well on all sides with the salt and pepper. Place the riblets in the air fryer basket and cook for 10 minutes, flipping halfway through.

3. While the riblets cook, mix all the sauce ingredients together in a 6-inch pie pan.

4. Remove the riblets from the air fryer and place them in the pie pan with the sauce. Stir to coat the riblets in the sauce. Transfer the pan to the air fryer and cook for 10 to 15 minutes, until the pork is cooked through and the internal temperature reaches 145°F.

5. Store leftovers in an airtight container in the refrigerator for up to 4 days. Reheat in a preheated 350°F air fryer for 5 minutes, or until heated through.

note: I was able to buy a rack of pork spare ribs already cut into riblets, but you may need to ask your butcher to cut a rack of spare ribs in half lengthwise to make sure these are the right size.

(per serving)   calories **319** | fat **26g** | protein **19g** | total carbs **3g** | fiber **0.3g**

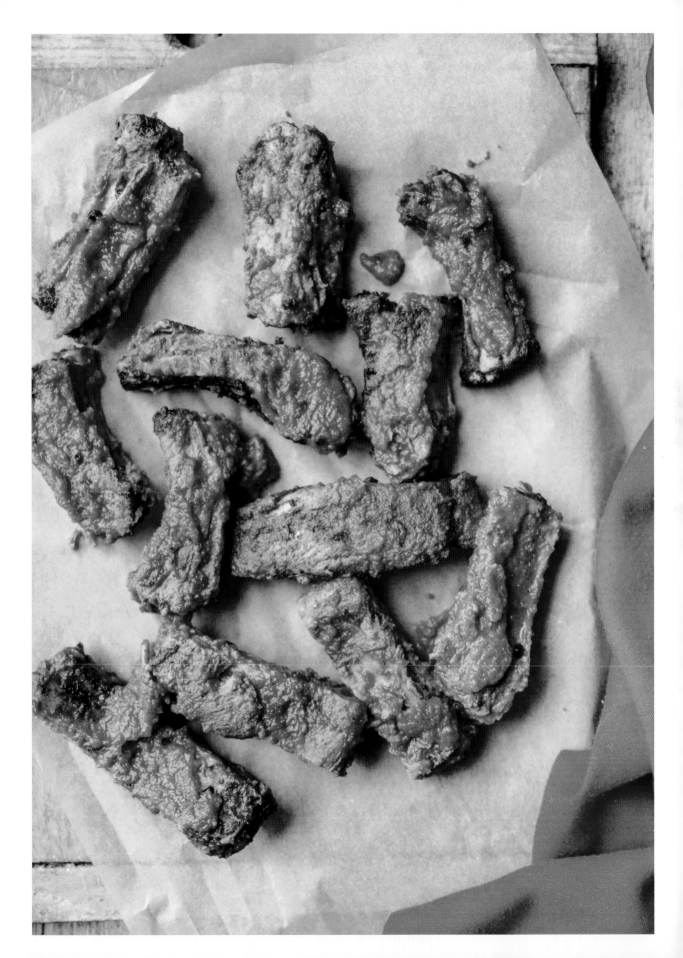

Dry Rub Baby Back Ribs

yield: 2 servings   *prep time:* 5 minutes   *cook time:* 35 minutes

2 teaspoons fine sea salt

1 teaspoon ground black pepper

2 teaspoons smoked paprika

1 teaspoon garlic powder

1 teaspoon onion powder

½ teaspoon chili powder
(optional, for a spicy kick)

1 rack baby back ribs, cut in half
crosswise

1. Spray the air fryer basket with avocado oil. Preheat the air fryer to 350°F.

2. In a small bowl, combine the salt, pepper, and seasonings. Season the ribs on all sides with the seasoning mixture.

3. Place the ribs in the air fryer basket and cook for 15 minutes, then flip the ribs over and cook for another 15 to 20 minutes, until the ribs are cooked through and the internal temperature reaches 145°F.

4. Store leftovers in an airtight container in the refrigerator for up to 4 days. Reheat in a preheated 350°F air fryer for 5 minutes, or until heated through.

(per serving)   calories **515** | fat **40g** | protein **37g** | total carbs **3g** | fiber **1g**

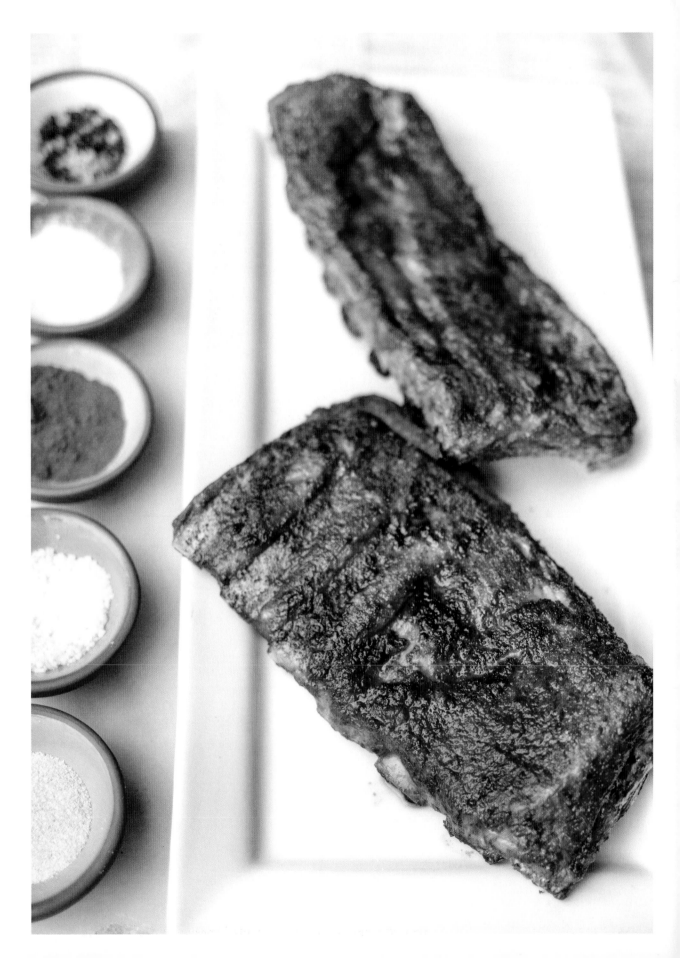

Bacon-Wrapped Stuffed Pork Chops

yield: 4 servings *prep time:* 10 minutes *cook time:* 20 minutes

4 (1-inch-thick) boneless pork chops

2 (5.2-ounce) packages Boursin cheese (or Kite Hill brand chive cream cheese style spread, softened, for dairy-free) (see Notes)

8 slices thin-cut bacon

notes: If you can't find Boursin cheese, you can use cream cheese and add 2 tablespoons of chopped fresh chives.

Try serving this dish with Garlic and Thyme Mushrooms (page 99)—they go great together!

1. Spray the air fryer basket with avocado oil. Preheat the air fryer to 400°F.

2. Place one of the chops on a cutting board. With a sharp knife held parallel to the cutting board, make a 1-inch-wide incision on the top edge of the chop. Carefully cut into the chop to form a large pocket, leaving a ½-inch border along the sides and bottom. Repeat with the other 3 chops.

3. Snip the corner of a large resealable plastic bag to form a ¾-inch hole. Place the Boursin cheese in the bag and pipe the cheese into the pockets in the chops, dividing the cheese evenly among them.

4. Wrap 2 slices of bacon around each chop and secure the ends with toothpicks. Place the bacon-wrapped chops in the air fryer basket and cook for 10 minutes, then flip the chops and cook for another 8 to 10 minutes, until the bacon is crisp, the chops are cooked through, and the internal temperature reaches 145°F.

5. Store leftovers in an airtight container in the refrigerator for up to 3 days. Reheat in a preheated 400°F air fryer for 5 minutes, or until warmed through.

(per serving)   calories **578** | fat **45g** | protein **37g** | total carbs **16g** | fiber **1g**

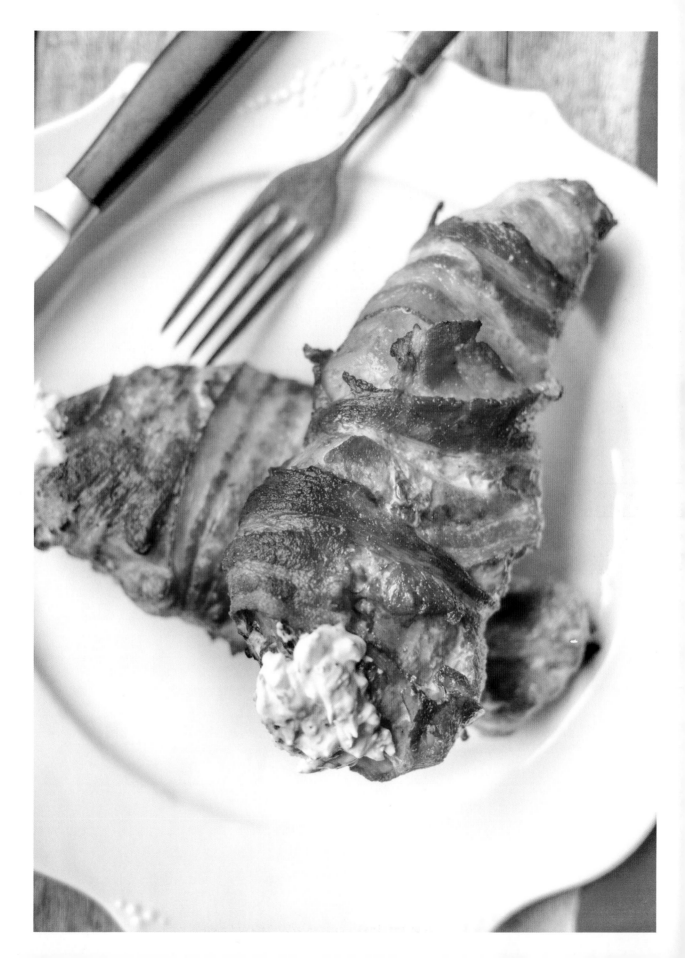

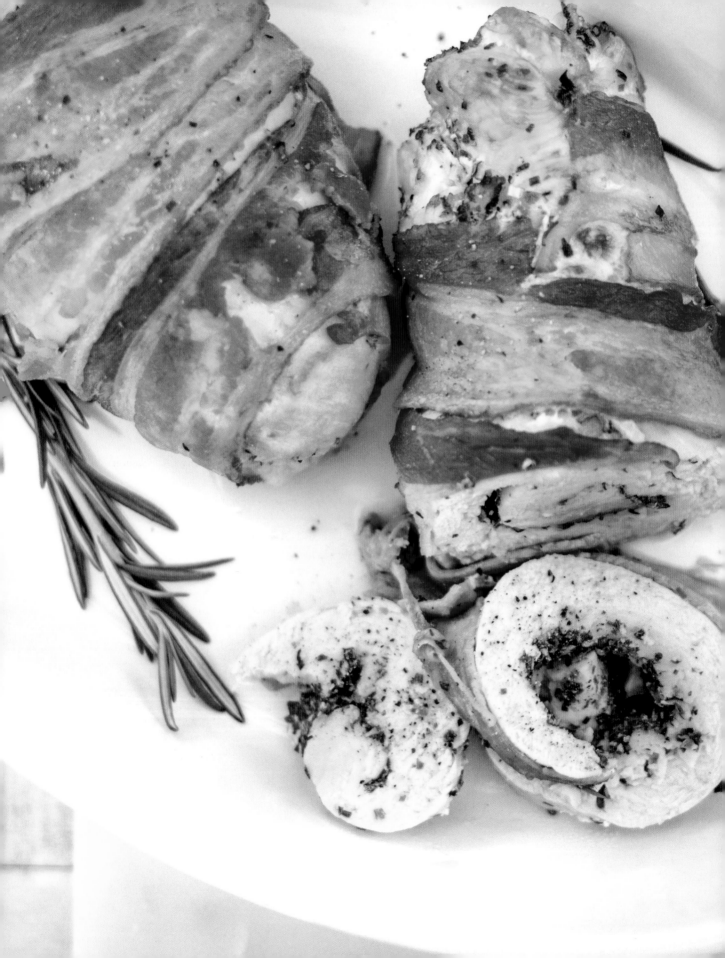

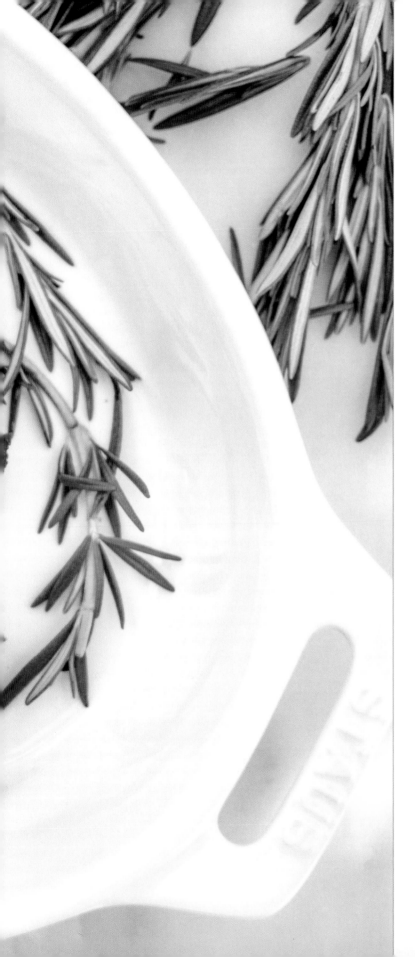

Poultry

Chicken Kiev

yield: 4 servings   *prep time:* 15 minutes   *cook time:* 25 minutes

option   KETO

1 cup (2 sticks) unsalted butter, softened (or butter-flavored coconut oil for dairy-free)

2 tablespoons lemon juice

2 tablespoons plus 1 teaspoon chopped fresh parsley leaves, divided, plus more for garnish

2 tablespoons chopped fresh tarragon leaves

3 cloves garlic, minced

1 teaspoon fine sea salt, divided

4 (4-ounce) boneless, skinless chicken breasts

2 large eggs

2 cups pork dust (see page 19)

1 teaspoon ground black pepper

Sprig of fresh parsley, for garnish

Lemon slices, for serving

1. Spray the air fryer basket with avocado oil. Preheat the air fryer to 350°F.

2. In a medium-sized bowl, combine the butter, lemon juice, 2 tablespoons of the parsley, the tarragon, garlic, and ¼ teaspoon of the salt. Cover and place in the fridge to harden for 7 minutes.

3. While the butter mixture chills, place one of the chicken breasts on a cutting board. With a sharp knife held parallel to the cutting board, make a 1-inch-wide incision at the top of the breast. Carefully cut into the breast to form a large pocket, leaving a ½-inch border along the sides and bottom. Repeat with the other 3 breasts.

4. Stuff one-quarter of the butter mixture into each chicken breast and secure the openings with toothpicks.

5. Beat the eggs in a small shallow dish. In another shallow dish, combine the pork dust, the remaining 1 teaspoon of parsley, the remaining ¾ teaspoon of salt, and the pepper.

6. One at a time, dip the chicken breasts in the egg, shake off the excess egg, and dredge the breasts in the pork dust mixture. Use your hands to press the pork dust onto each breast to form a nice crust. If you desire a thicker coating, dip it again in the egg and pork dust. As you finish, spray each coated chicken breast with avocado oil and place it in the air fryer basket.

7. Cook the chicken in the air fryer for 15 minutes, flip the breasts, and cook for another 10 minutes, or until the internal temperature of the chicken is 165°F and the crust is golden brown.

8. Serve garnished with chopped fresh parsley and a parsley sprig, with lemon slices on the side.

9. Store leftovers in an airtight container in the refrigerator for up to 4 days or in the freezer for up to a month. Reheat in a preheated 350°F air fryer for 5 minutes, or until heated through.

(per serving)   calories **801** | fat **64g** | protein **51g** | total carbs **3g** | fiber **1g**

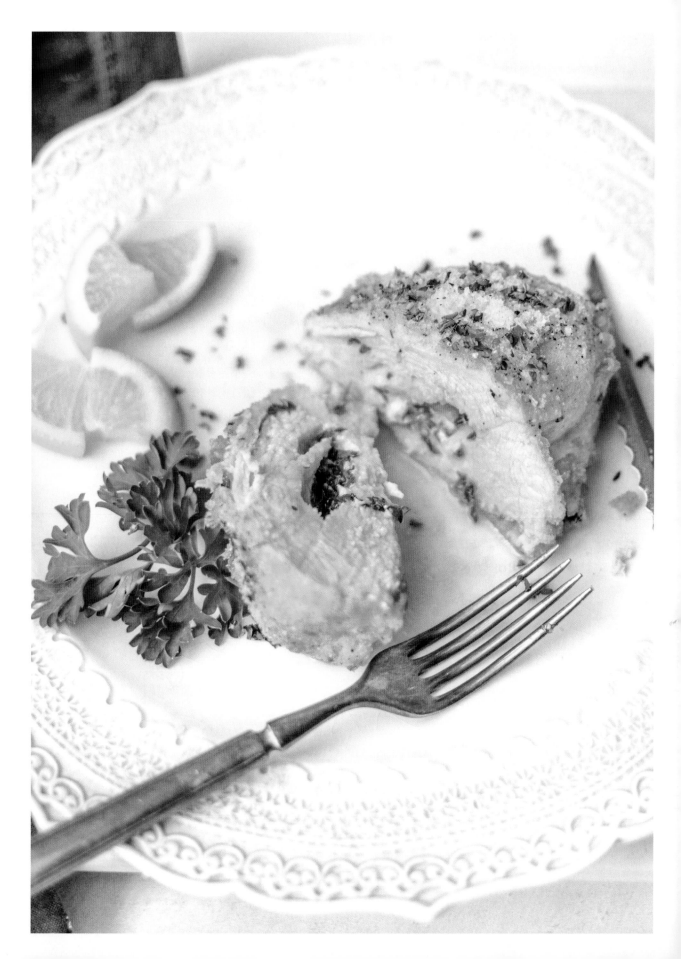

Chicken Cordon Bleu Meatballs

yield: 4 servings   *prep time:* 10 minutes   *cook time:* 15 minutes

KETO

MEATBALLS:

½ pound ground chicken

½ pound ham, diced

½ cup finely grated Swiss cheese (about 2 ounces)

¼ cup chopped onions

3 cloves garlic, minced

1½ teaspoons fine sea salt

1 teaspoon ground black pepper, plus more for garnish if desired

1 large egg, beaten

DIJON SAUCE:

¼ cup chicken broth, hot

3 tablespoons Dijon mustard

2 tablespoons lemon juice

¾ teaspoon fine sea salt

¼ teaspoon ground black pepper

Chopped fresh thyme leaves, for garnish (optional)

1. Spray the air fryer basket with avocado oil. Preheat the air fryer to 390°F.

2. In a large bowl, mix all the ingredients for the meatballs with your hands until well combined. Shape the meat mixture into about twelve 1½-inch balls. Place the meatballs in the air fryer basket, leaving space between them, and cook for 15 minutes, or until cooked through and the internal temperature reaches 165°F.

3. While the meatballs cook, make the sauce: In a small mixing bowl, stir together all the sauce ingredients until well combined.

4. Pour the sauce into a serving dish and place the meatballs on top. Garnish with ground black pepper and fresh thyme leaves, if desired.

5. Store leftover meatballs in an airtight container in the refrigerator for up to 5 days or in the freezer for up to a month. Reheat in a preheated 350°F air fryer for 4 minutes, or until heated through.

(per serving)   calories **288** | fat **15g** | protein **31g** | total carbs **5g** | fiber **0.5g**

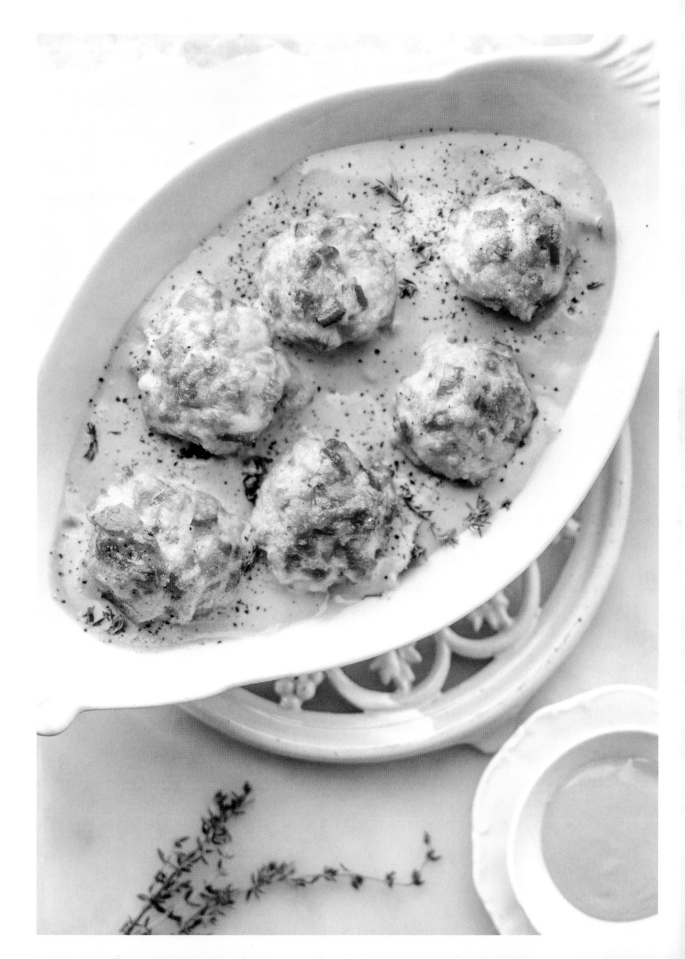

Buffalo Chicken Drumsticks

yield: 8 servings   *prep time:* 10 minutes, plus 2 hours to marinate   *cook time:* 25 minutes

1 cup dill pickle juice

2 pounds chicken drumsticks

2 teaspoons fine sea salt

WING SAUCE:

⅓ cup hot sauce

¼ cup unsalted butter, melted

1 tablespoon lime juice

½ teaspoon fine sea salt

⅛ teaspoon garlic powder

FOR SERVING:

½ cup Blue Cheese Dressing (page 54) or Ranch Dressing (page 68)

Celery sticks

busy family tip: You can skip the step of marinating the chicken, but it adds a lot of flavor.

1. Place the dill pickle juice in a large shallow dish and add the chicken. Spoon the juice over the chicken, cover, and place in the fridge to marinate for 2 hours or overnight.

2. Spray the air fryer basket with avocado oil. Preheat the air fryer to 400°F.

3. Pat the chicken dry and season it well with the salt. Cook in the air fryer for 20 minutes, or until the internal temperature reaches 165°F, flipping after 15 minutes.

4. While the chicken cooks, make the wing sauce: In a large mixing bowl, stir together all the sauce ingredients until well combined.

5. Remove the drumsticks from the air fryer and place them in the bowl with the sauce. Coat the drumsticks well with the sauce, then use tongs or a slotted spoon to return them to the air fryer basket and cook for 5 minutes more. Serve with any extra wing sauce, blue cheese dressing, and celery sticks.

6. Store extra drumsticks in an airtight container in the fridge for up to 4 days or in the freezer for up to a month. Reheat in a preheated 350°F air fryer for 5 minutes, then increase the temperature to 400°F and cook for 3 to 5 minutes more, until warm and crispy.

(per serving)   calories **472** | fat **34g** | protein **38g** | total carbs **1g** | fiber **0.3g**

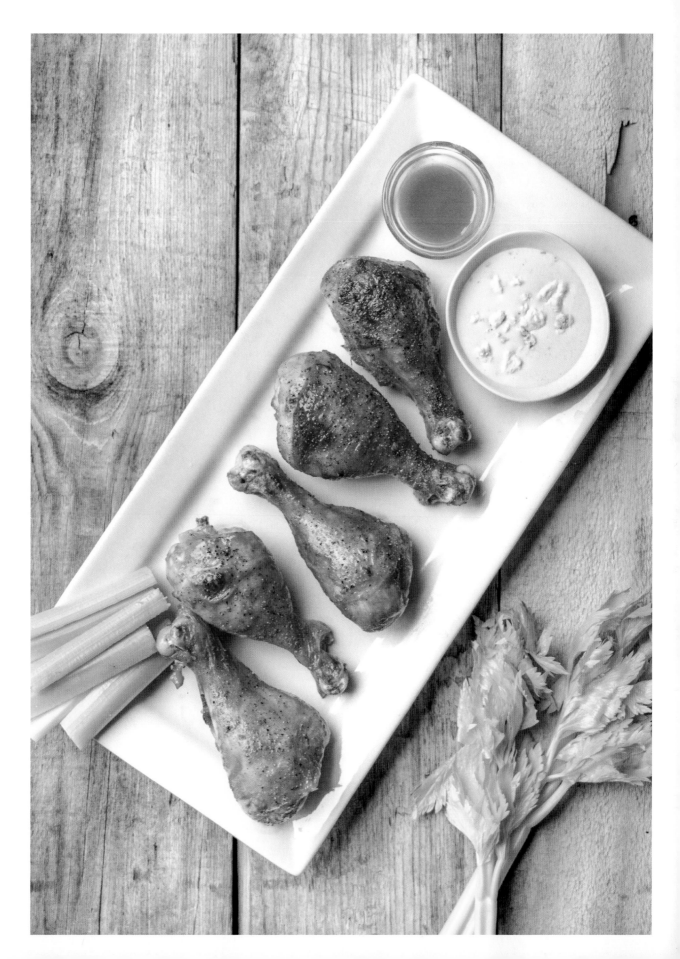

Sesame Turkey Balls in Lettuce Cups

yield: 6 servings   *prep time:* 10 minutes   *cook time:* 15 minutes

MEATBALLS:

2 pounds ground turkey

2 large eggs, beaten

¾ cup finely chopped button mushrooms

¼ cup finely chopped green onions, plus more for garnish if desired

2 tablespoons Swerve confectioners'-style sweetener or equivalent amount of liquid or powdered sweetener (see page 18)

2 teaspoons peeled and grated fresh ginger

2 teaspoons toasted sesame oil

1½ teaspoons wheat-free tamari, or 2 tablespoons coconut aminos

1 clove garlic, smashed to a paste

SAUCE:

½ cup chicken broth

⅓ cup Swerve confectioners'-style sweetener or equivalent amount of liquid or powdered sweetener (see page 18)

2 tablespoons toasted sesame oil

2 tablespoons tomato sauce

2 tablespoons wheat-free tamari, or ½ cup coconut aminos

1 tablespoon lime juice

¼ teaspoon peeled and grated fresh ginger

1 clove garlic, smashed to a paste

Boston lettuce leaves, for serving

Sliced red chiles, for garnish (optional)

Toasted sesame seeds, for garnish (optional)

1. Preheat the air fryer to 350°F.

2. Place all the ingredients for the meatballs in a large bowl and, using your hands, mix them together until well combined. Shape the mixture into about twelve 1½-inch meatballs and place them in a pie pan that will fit in the air fryer, leaving space between them.

3. Make the sauce: In a medium-sized bowl, stir together all the sauce ingredients until well combined. Pour the sauce over the meatballs.

4. Place the pan in the air fryer and cook for 15 minutes, or until the internal temperature of the meatballs reaches 165°F, flipping after 6 minutes.

5. To serve, lay several lettuce leaves on a serving plate and place several meatballs on top. Garnish with sliced red chiles, green onions, and/or sesame seeds, if desired.

6. Store leftovers in an airtight container in the refrigerator for up to 4 days or in the freezer for up to a month. Reheat in a preheated 350°F air fryer for 5 minutes, or until warmed through.

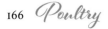

(per serving)   calories **322** | fat **19g** | protein **32g** | total carbs **2g** | fiber **0.3g**

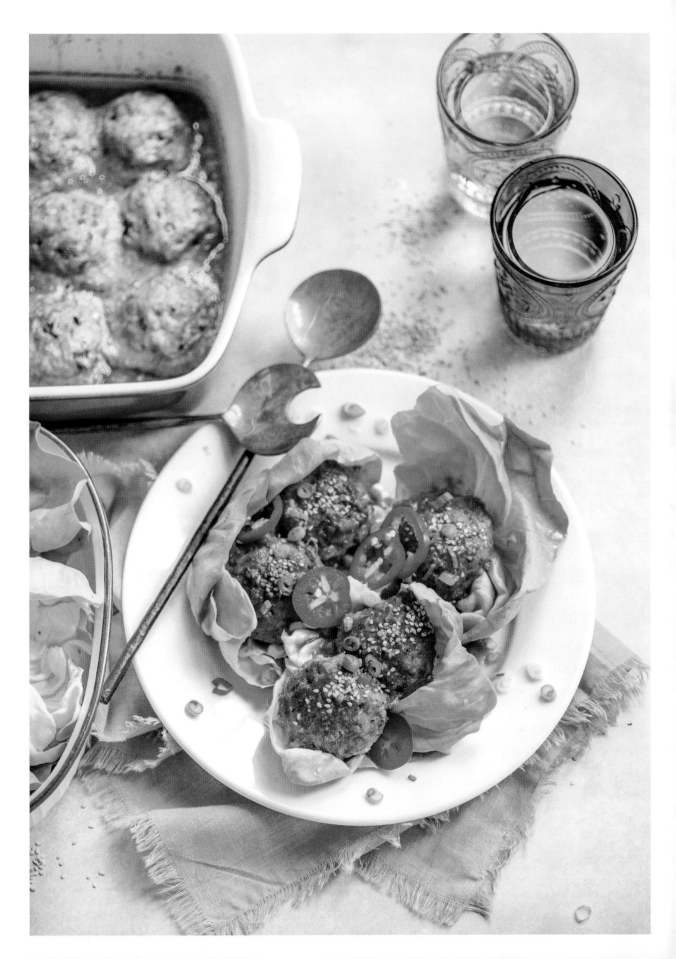

Porchetta-Style Chicken Breasts

yield: 4 servings   *prep time:* 10 minutes   *cook time:* 15 minutes

½ cup fresh parsley leaves

¼ cup roughly chopped fresh chives

4 cloves garlic, peeled

2 tablespoons lemon juice

3 teaspoons fine sea salt

1 teaspoon dried rubbed sage

1 teaspoon fresh rosemary leaves

1 teaspoon ground fennel

½ teaspoon red pepper flakes

4 (4-ounce) boneless, skinless chicken breasts, pounded to ¼ inch thick (see Tip)

8 slices bacon

Sprigs of fresh rosemary, for garnish (optional)

1. Spray the air fryer basket with avocado oil. Preheat the air fryer to 340°F.

2. Place the parsley, chives, garlic, lemon juice, salt, sage, rosemary, fennel, and red pepper flakes in a food processor and puree until a smooth paste forms.

3. Place the chicken breasts on a cutting board and rub the paste all over the tops. With a short end facing you, roll each breast up like a jelly roll to make a log and secure it with toothpicks.

4. Wrap 2 slices of bacon around each chicken breast log to cover the entire breast. Secure the bacon with toothpicks.

5. Place the chicken breast logs in the air fryer basket and cook for 5 minutes, flip the logs over, and cook for another 5 minutes. Increase the heat to 390°F and cook until the bacon is crisp, about 5 minutes more.

6. Remove the toothpicks and garnish with fresh rosemary sprigs, if desired, before serving. Store leftovers in an airtight container in the refrigerator for up to 4 days or in the freezer for up to a month. Reheat in a preheated 350°F air fryer for 5 minutes, then increase the heat to 390°F and cook for 2 minutes to crisp the bacon.

tip: I asked my butcher to pound out the chicken breasts to the desired thickness, saving me time and making this recipe even easier!

(per serving)   calories **468** | fat **25g** | protein **56g** | total carbs **3g** | fiber **1g**

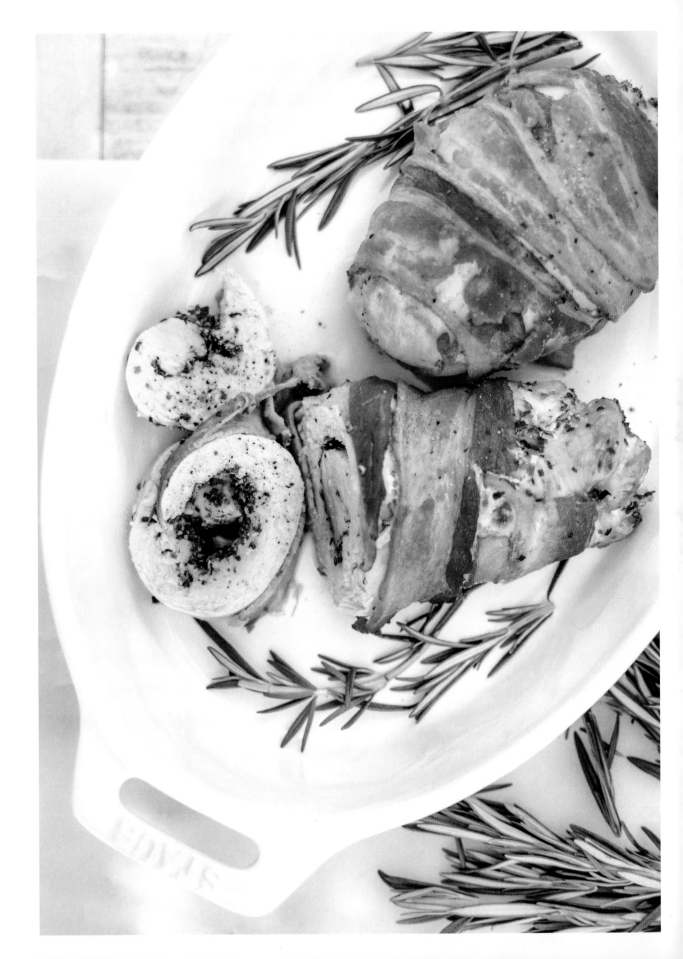

Easy Thanksgiving Turkey Breast

yield: 4 servings   *prep time:* 5 minutes   *cook time:* 30 minutes

1½ teaspoons fine sea salt

1 teaspoon ground black pepper

1 teaspoon chopped fresh rosemary leaves

1 teaspoon chopped fresh sage

1 teaspoon chopped fresh tarragon

1 teaspoon chopped fresh thyme leaves

1 (2-pound) turkey breast

3 tablespoons ghee or unsalted butter, melted

3 tablespoons Dijon mustard

1. Spray the air fryer with avocado oil. Preheat the air fryer to 390°F.

2. In a small bowl, stir together the salt, pepper, and herbs until well combined. Season the turkey breast generously on all sides with the seasoning.

3. In another small bowl, stir together the ghee and Dijon. Brush the ghee mixture on all sides of the turkey breast.

4. Place the turkey breast in the air fryer basket and cook for 30 minutes, or until the internal temperature reaches 165°F. Transfer the breast to a cutting board and allow it to rest for 10 minutes before cutting it into ½-inch-thick slices.

5. Store leftovers in an airtight container in the refrigerator for up to 4 days or in the freezer for up to a month. Reheat in a preheated 350°F air fryer for 4 minutes, or until warmed through.

(per serving) calories **388** | fat **18g** | protein **50g** | total carbs **1g** | fiber **0.3g**

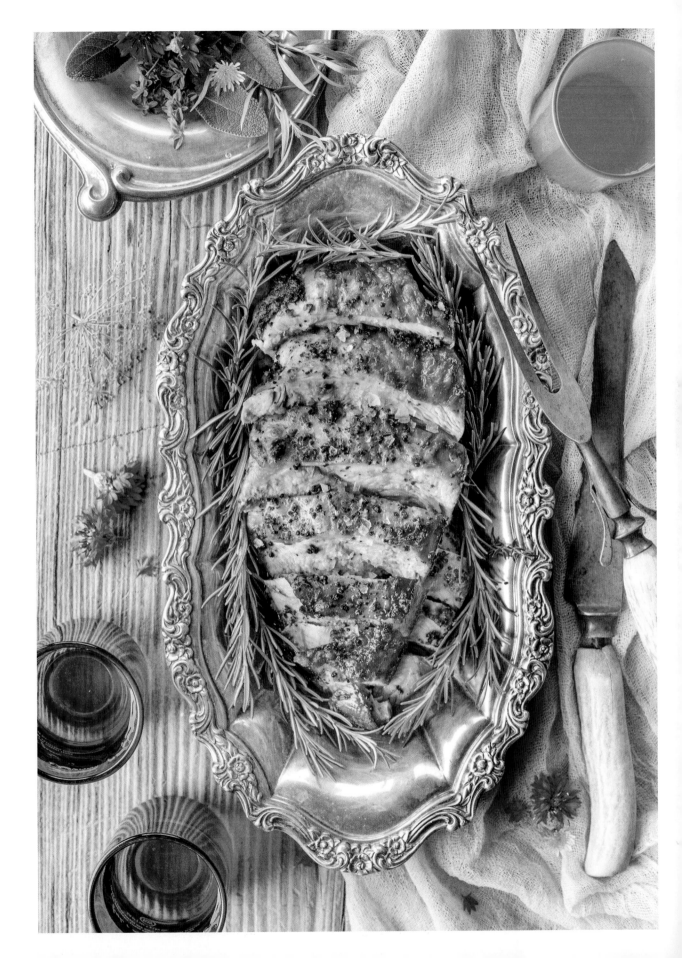

Chicken Paillard

yield: 2 servings *prep time:* 10 minutes *cook time:* 10 minutes

KETO

2 large eggs, room temperature

1 tablespoon water

½ cup powdered Parmesan cheese (about 1½ ounces; see page 19) or pork dust (see page 19)

2 teaspoons dried thyme leaves

1 teaspoon ground black pepper

2 (5-ounce) boneless, skinless chicken breasts, pounded to ½ inch thick (see Tip, page 168)

LEMON BUTTER SAUCE:

2 tablespoons unsalted butter, melted

2 teaspoons lemon juice

¼ teaspoon finely chopped fresh thyme leaves, plus more for garnish

⅛ teaspoon fine sea salt

Lemon slices, for serving

1. Spray the air fryer basket with avocado oil. Preheat the air fryer to 390°F.

2. Beat the eggs in a shallow dish, then add the water and stir well.

3. In a separate shallow dish, mix together the Parmesan, thyme, and pepper until well combined.

4. One at a time, dip the chicken breasts in the eggs and let any excess drip off, then dredge both sides of the chicken in the Parmesan mixture. As you finish, set the coated chicken in the air fryer basket.

5. Cook the chicken in the air fryer for 5 minutes, then flip the chicken and cook for another 5 minutes, or until cooked through and the internal temperature reaches 165°F.

6. While the chicken cooks, make the lemon butter sauce: In a small bowl, mix together all the sauce ingredients until well combined.

7. Plate the chicken and pour the sauce over it. Garnish with chopped fresh thyme and serve with lemon slices.

8. Store leftovers in an airtight container in the refrigerator for up to 4 days. Reheat in a preheated 390°F air fryer for 5 minutes, or until heated through.

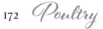

(per serving) calories **526** | fat **33g** | protein **53g** | total carbs **3g** | fiber **1g**

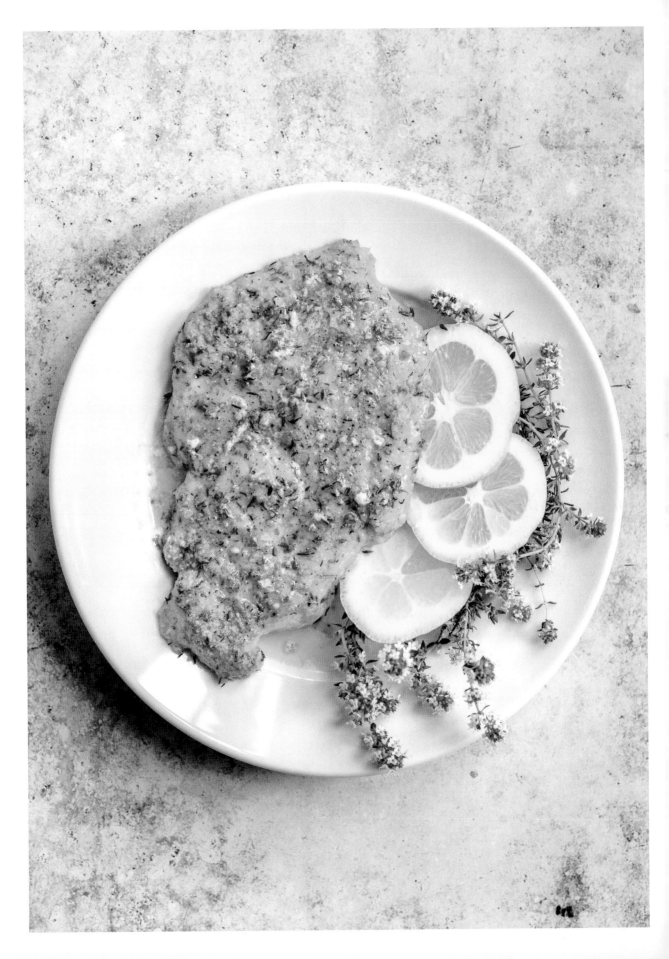

General Tso's Chicken

yield: 4 servings *prep time:* 10 minutes *cook time:* 20 minutes

1 pound boneless, skinless chicken breasts or thighs, cut into 1-inch cubes

Fine sea salt and ground black pepper

GENERAL TSO'S SAUCE:

½ cup chicken broth

⅓ cup Swerve confectioners'-style sweetener or equivalent amount of liquid or powdered sweetener (see page 18)

¼ cup coconut vinegar or unseasoned rice vinegar

¼ cup thinly sliced green onions, plus more for garnish if desired

1 tablespoon plus 1¼ teaspoons wheat-free tamari, or ¼ cup coconut aminos

3 small dried red chiles, chopped

1 clove garlic, minced

1½ teaspoons grated fresh ginger

1 teaspoon toasted sesame oil

¼ teaspoon guar gum (optional; see Tips)

FOR SERVING (OPTIONAL):

Fried Cauliflower Rice (page 98)

Sautéed broccoli rabe

FOR GARNISH (OPTIONAL):

Diced red chiles

Red pepper flakes

Sesame seeds

1. Preheat the air fryer to 400°F.

2. Very lightly season the chicken on all sides with salt and pepper (the sauce will add seasoning). Place the chicken in a single layer in a pie pan that fits in the air fryer and cook for 5 minutes.

3. While the chicken cooks, make the sauce: In a small bowl, stir together all the sauce ingredients except the guar gum until well combined. Sift in the guar gum (if using) and whisk until well combined.

4. Pour the sauce over the chicken and, stirring every 5 minutes, cook for another 12 to 15 minutes, until the sauce is bubbly and thick and the chicken is cooked through and the internal temperature reaches 165°F.

5. If you want the sauce to be even thicker and more flavorful, remove the chicken and return the sauce to the air fryer to cook for an additional 5 to 10 minutes.

6. Transfer the chicken to a large bowl. Serve with fried cauliflower rice and sautéed broccoli rabe, if desired, and garnish with diced red chiles, sliced green onions, red pepper flakes, and sesame seeds, if desired.

7. Store leftovers in an airtight container in the refrigerator for up to 4 days. Reheat in a preheated 375°F air fryer for 5 minutes, or until heated through.

tips: *If you're using homemade chicken broth, you probably won't need the guar gum, but it's a nice thickener for store-bought broth.*

This recipe makes a lot of sauce. If you have extra, it tastes delicious poured over Fried Cauliflower Rice (page 98).

(per serving) calories **254** | fat **10g** | protein **34g** | total carbs **5g** | fiber **1g**

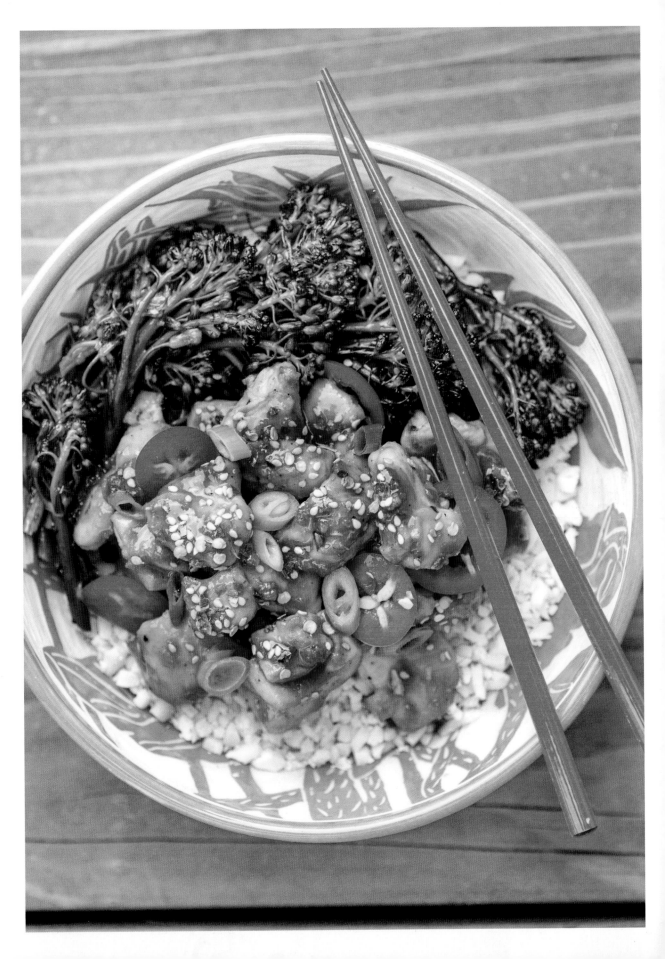

Chicken Strips with Satay Sauce

yield: 4 servings *prep time:* 5 minutes *cook time:* 10 minutes

option KETO

4 (6-ounce) boneless, skinless chicken breasts, sliced into 16 (1-inch) strips

1 teaspoon fine sea salt

1 teaspoon paprika

SAUCE:

¼ cup creamy almond butter (or sunflower seed butter for nut-free)

2 tablespoons chicken broth

1½ tablespoons coconut vinegar or unseasoned rice vinegar

1 clove garlic, minced

1 teaspoon peeled and minced fresh ginger

½ teaspoon hot sauce

⅛ teaspoon stevia glycerite, or 2 to 3 drops liquid stevia

FOR GARNISH/SERVING (OPTIONAL):

¼ cup chopped cilantro leaves

Red pepper flakes

Sea salt flakes

Thinly sliced red, orange, and yellow bell peppers

special equipment: x16

16 wooden or bamboo skewers, soaked in water for 15 minutes

1. Spray the air fryer basket with avocado oil. Preheat the air fryer to 400°F.

2. Thread the chicken strips onto the skewers. Season on all sides with the salt and paprika. Place the chicken skewers in the air fryer basket and cook for 5 minutes, flip, and cook for another 5 minutes, until the chicken is cooked through and the internal temperature reaches 165°F.

3. While the chicken skewers cook, make the sauce: In a medium-sized bowl, stir together all the sauce ingredients until well combined. Taste and adjust the sweetness and heat to your liking.

4. Garnish the chicken with cilantro, red pepper flakes, and salt flakes, if desired, and serve with sliced bell peppers, if desired. Serve the sauce on the side.

5. Store leftovers in an airtight container in the fridge for up to 4 days or in the freezer for up to a month. Reheat in a preheated 350°F air fryer for 3 minutes per side, or until heated through.

(per serving) calories **359** | fat **16g** | protein **49g** | total carbs **2g** | fiber **1g**

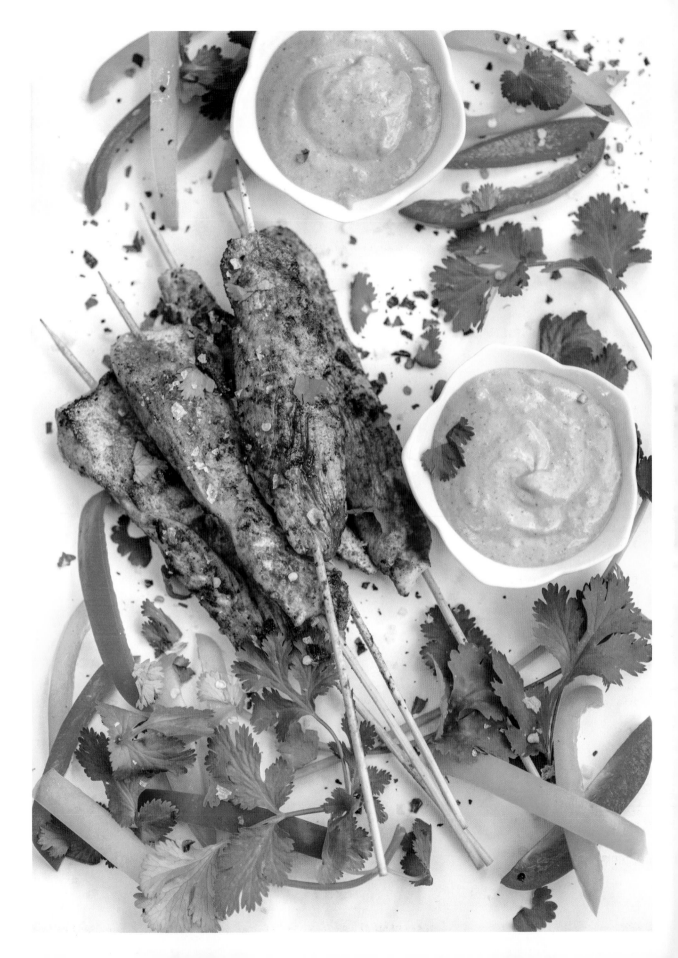

Bacon Lovers' Stuffed Chicken

yield: 4 servings   *prep time:* 10 minutes   *cook time:* 20 minutes

option   KETO

4 (5-ounce) boneless, skinless chicken breasts, pounded to ¼ inch thick (see Tip, page 168)

2 (5.2-ounce) packages Boursin cheese (or Kite Hill brand chive cream cheese style spread, softened, for dairy-free) (see Tip)

8 slices thin-cut bacon or beef bacon

Sprig of fresh cilantro, for garnish (optional)

1. Spray the air fryer basket with avocado oil. Preheat the air fryer to 400°F.

2. Place one of the chicken breasts on a cutting board. With a sharp knife held parallel to the cutting board, make a 1-inch-wide incision at the top of the breast. Carefully cut into the breast to form a large pocket, leaving a ½-inch border along the sides and bottom. Repeat with the other 3 chicken breasts.

3. Snip the corner of a large resealable plastic bag to form a ¾-inch hole. Place the Boursin cheese in the bag and pipe the cheese into the pockets in the chicken breasts, dividing the cheese evenly among them.

4. Wrap 2 slices of bacon around each chicken breast and secure the ends with toothpicks. Place the bacon-wrapped chicken in the air fryer basket and cook until the bacon is crisp and the chicken's internal temperature reaches 165°F, about 18 to 20 minutes, flipping after 10 minutes. Garnish with a sprig of cilantro before serving, if desired.

5. Store leftovers in an airtight container in the refrigerator for up to 4 days. Reheat in a preheated 400°F air fryer for 5 minutes, or until warmed through.

tip: If you can't find Boursin cheese, you can use cream cheese and add 2 tablespoons of chopped fresh chives.

(per serving)   calories **686** | fat **51g** | protein **52g** | total carbs **2g** | fiber **0g**

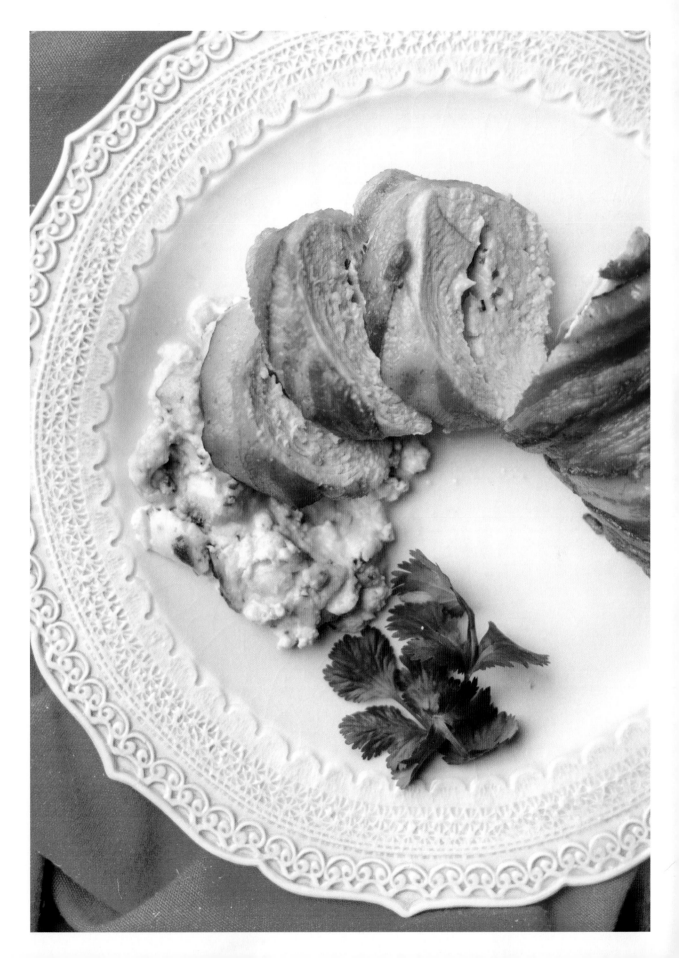

Chicken Pesto Parmigiana

yield: 4 servings   *prep time:* 10 minutes   *cook time:* 23 minutes

option   KETO

2 large eggs

1 tablespoon water

Fine sea salt and ground black pepper

1 cup powdered Parmesan cheese (about 3 ounces) (see page 19)

2 teaspoons Italian seasoning

4 (5-ounce) boneless, skinless chicken breasts or thighs, pounded to ¼ inch thick (see Note; see Tip, page 168)

1 cup pesto (page 202)

1 cup shredded mozzarella cheese (about 4 ounces)

Finely chopped fresh basil, for garnish (optional)

Grape tomatoes, halved, for serving (optional)

1. Spray the air fryer basket with avocado oil. Preheat the air fryer to 400°F.

2. Crack the eggs into a shallow baking dish, add the water and a pinch each of salt and pepper, and whisk to combine. In another shallow baking dish, stir together the Parmesan and Italian seasoning until well combined.

3. Season the chicken breasts well on both sides with salt and pepper. Dip one chicken breast in the eggs and let any excess drip off, then dredge both sides of the breast in the Parmesan mixture. Spray the breast with avocado oil and place it in the air fryer basket. Repeat with the remaining 3 chicken breasts.

4. Cook the chicken in the air fryer for 20 minutes, or until the internal temperature reaches 165°F and the breading is golden brown, flipping halfway through.

5. Dollop each chicken breast with ¼ cup of the pesto and top with the mozzarella. Return the breasts to the air fryer and cook for 3 minutes, or until the cheese is melted. Garnish with basil and serve with halved grape tomatoes on the side, if desired.

6. Store leftovers in an airtight container in the refrigerator for up to 4 days. Reheat in a preheated 400°F air fryer for 5 minutes, or until warmed through.

note: You can use either chicken breasts or thighs, but the coating sticks better to chicken breasts: the additional fat in thighs causes the coating to slide off.

(per serving, with breasts) calories **558** | fat **43g** | protein **40g** | total carbs **4g** | fiber **1g**

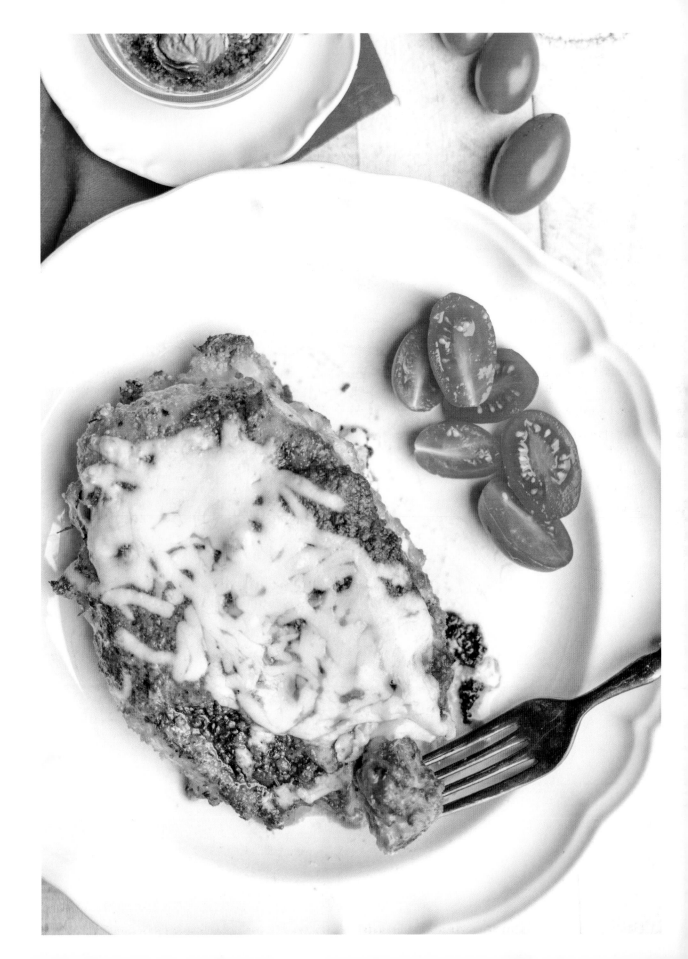

Crispy Taco Chicken

yield: 4 servings   *prep time:* 10 minutes   *cook time:* 23 minutes

2 large eggs

1 tablespoon water

Fine sea salt and ground black pepper

1 cup pork dust (see page 19)

1 teaspoon ground cumin

1 teaspoon smoked paprika

4 (5-ounce) boneless, skinless chicken breasts or thighs, pounded to ¼ inch thick (see Note; see Tip, page 168)

1 cup salsa

1 cup shredded Monterey Jack cheese (about 4 ounces) (omit for dairy-free)

Sprig of fresh cilantro, for garnish (optional)

1. Spray the air fryer basket with avocado oil. Preheat the air fryer to 400°F.

2. Crack the eggs into a shallow baking dish, add the water and a pinch each of salt and pepper, and whisk to combine. In another shallow baking dish, stir together the pork dust, cumin, and paprika until well combined.

3. Season the chicken breasts well on both sides with salt and pepper. Dip 1 chicken breast in the eggs and let any excess drip off, then dredge both sides of the chicken breast in the pork dust mixture. Spray the breast with avocado oil and place it in the air fryer basket. Repeat with the remaining 3 chicken breasts.

4. Cook the chicken in the air fryer for 20 minutes, or until the internal temperature reaches 165°F and the breading is golden brown, flipping halfway through.

5. Dollop each chicken breast with ¼ cup of the salsa and top with ¼ cup of the cheese. Return the breasts to the air fryer and cook for 3 minutes, or until the cheese is melted. Garnish with cilantro before serving, if desired.

6. Store leftovers in an airtight container in the refrigerator for up to 4 days. Reheat in a preheated 400°F air fryer for 5 minutes, or until warmed through.

note: *You can use either chicken breasts or thighs, but the coating sticks better to chicken breasts: the additional fat in thighs causes the coating to slide off.*

(per serving, with breasts) calories **486** | fat **29g** | protein **54g** | total carbs **3g** | fiber **0.2g**

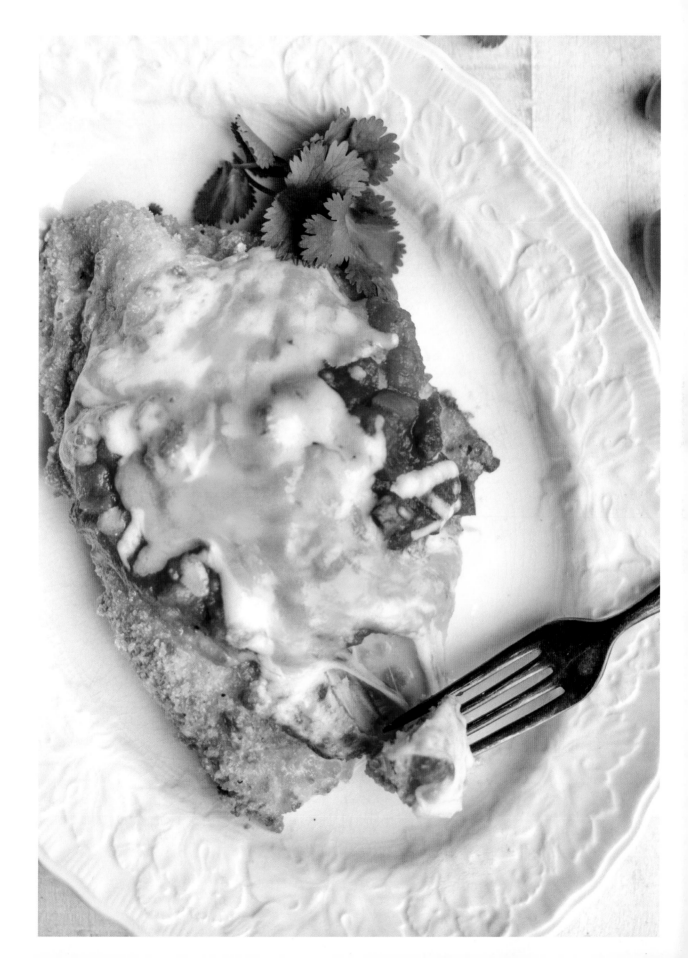

Thai Tacos with Peanut Sauce

yield: 4 servings   *prep time:* 10 minutes   *cook time:* 6 minutes

1 pound ground chicken

¼ cup diced onions (about 1 small onion)

2 cloves garlic, minced

¼ teaspoon fine sea salt

SAUCE:

¼ cup creamy peanut butter, room temperature

2 tablespoons chicken broth, plus more if needed

2 tablespoons lime juice

2 tablespoons grated fresh ginger

2 tablespoons wheat-free tamari or coconut aminos

1½ teaspoons hot sauce

5 drops liquid stevia (optional)

FOR SERVING:

2 small heads butter lettuce, leaves separated

Lime slices (optional)

FOR GARNISH (OPTIONAL):

Cilantro leaves

Shredded purple cabbage

Sliced green onions

1. Preheat the air fryer to 350°F.

2. Place the ground chicken, onions, garlic, and salt in a 6-inch pie pan or a dish that will fit in your air fryer. Break up the chicken with a spatula. Place in the air fryer and cook for 5 minutes, or until the chicken is browned and cooked through. Break up the chicken again into small crumbles.

3. Make the sauce: In a medium-sized bowl, stir together the peanut butter, broth, lime juice, ginger, tamari, hot sauce, and stevia (if using) until well combined. If the sauce is too thick, add another tablespoon or two of broth. Taste and add more hot sauce if desired.

4. Add half of the sauce to the pan with the chicken. Cook for another minute, until heated through, and stir well to combine.

5. Assemble the tacos: Place several lettuce leaves on a serving plate. Place a few tablespoons of the chicken mixture in each lettuce leaf and garnish with cilantro leaves, purple cabbage, and sliced green onions, if desired. Serve the remaining sauce on the side. Serve with lime slices, if desired.

6. Store leftover meat mixture in an airtight container in the refrigerator for up to 4 days; store leftover sauce, lettuce leaves, and garnishes separately. Reheat the meat mixture in a lightly greased pie pan in a preheated 350°F air fryer for 3 minutes, or until heated through.

(per serving)   calories **350** | fat **17g** | protein **39g** | total carbs **11g** | fiber **3g**

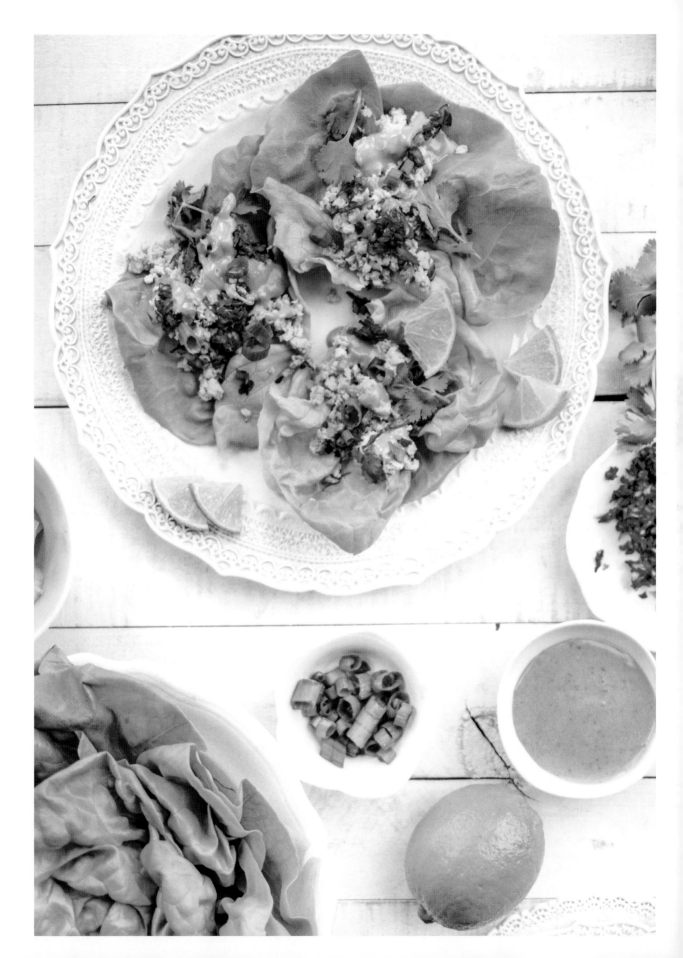

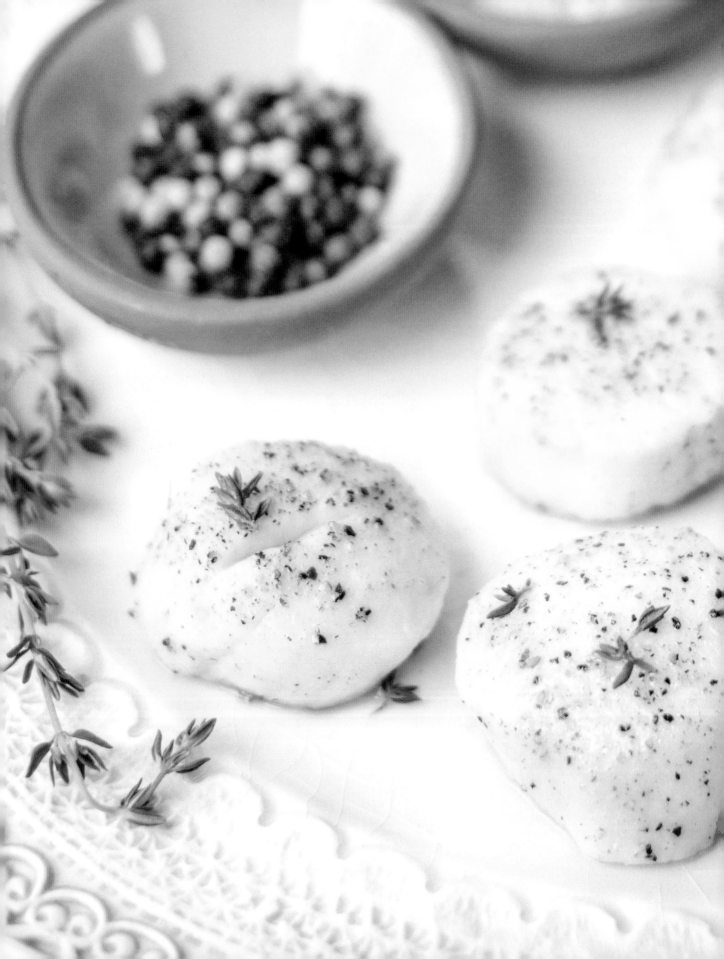

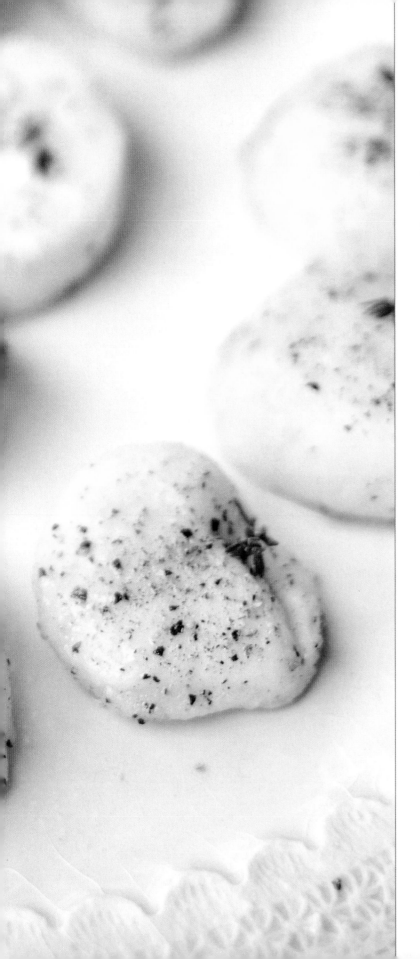

Fish and Seafood

Shrimp Scampi

yield: 4 servings   *prep time:* 5 minutes   *cook time:* 8 minutes

¼ cup unsalted butter (or butter-flavored coconut oil for dairy-free)

2 tablespoons fish stock or chicken broth

1 tablespoon lemon juice

2 cloves garlic, minced

2 tablespoons chopped fresh basil leaves

1 tablespoon chopped fresh parsley, plus more for garnish

1 teaspoon red pepper flakes

1 pound large shrimp, peeled and deveined, tails removed

Fresh basil sprigs, for garnish

1. Preheat the air fryer to 350° F.

2. Place the butter, fish stock, lemon juice, garlic, basil, parsley, and red pepper flakes in a 6 by 3-inch pan, stir to combine, and place in the air fryer. Cook for 3 minutes, or until fragrant and the garlic has softened.

3. Add the shrimp and stir to coat the shrimp in the sauce. Cook for 5 minutes, or until the shrimp are pink, stirring after 3 minutes. Garnish with fresh basil sprigs and chopped parsley before serving.

4. Store leftovers in an airtight container in the refrigerator for up to 4 days. Reheat in a preheated 400°F air fryer for about 3 minutes, until heated through.

(per serving)   calories **175** | fat **11g** | protein **18g** | total carbs **1g** | fiber **0.2g**

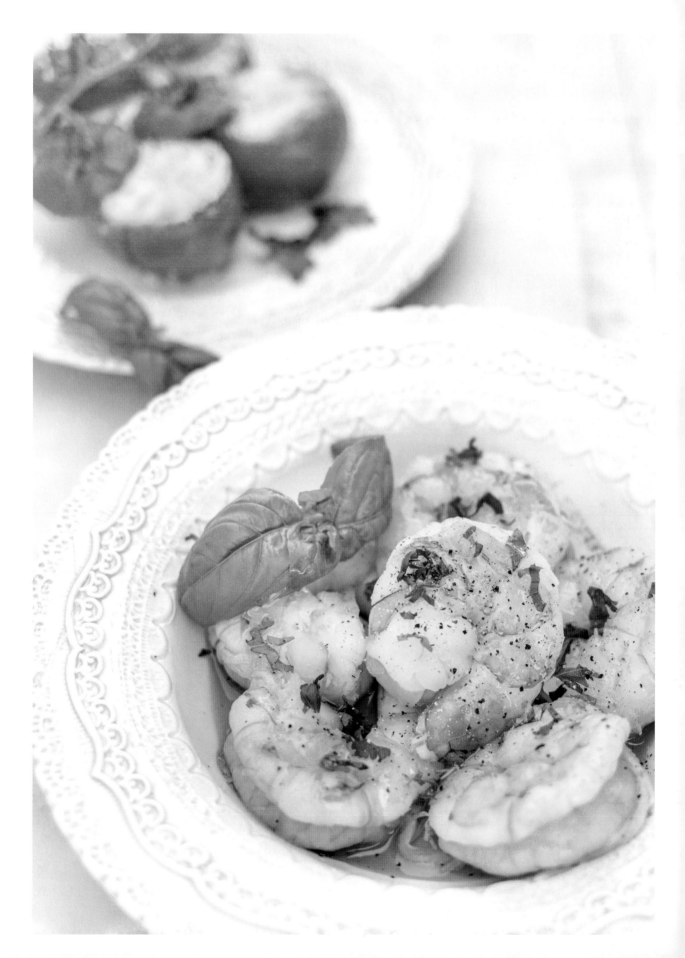

Simple Scallops

yield: 2 servings   *prep time:* 5 minutes   *cook time:* 4 minutes

12 medium sea scallops

1 teaspoon fine sea salt

¾ teaspoon ground black pepper, plus more for garnish if desired

Fresh thyme leaves, for garnish (optional)

1. Spray the air fryer basket with avocado oil. Preheat the air fryer to 390°F.

2. Rinse the scallops and pat completely dry. Spray avocado oil on the scallops and season them with the salt and pepper. Place them in the air fryer basket, spacing them apart (if you're using a smaller air fryer, work in batches if necessary). Cook for 2 minutes, then flip the scallops and cook for another 2 minutes, or until cooked through and no longer translucent. Garnish with ground black pepper and thyme leaves, if desired.

3. Best served fresh. Store leftovers in an airtight container in the fridge for up to 3 days. Reheat in a preheated 350°F air fryer for 2 minutes, or until heated through.

(per serving)   calories **106** | fat **2g** | protein **18g** | total carbs **3g** | fiber **0.2g**

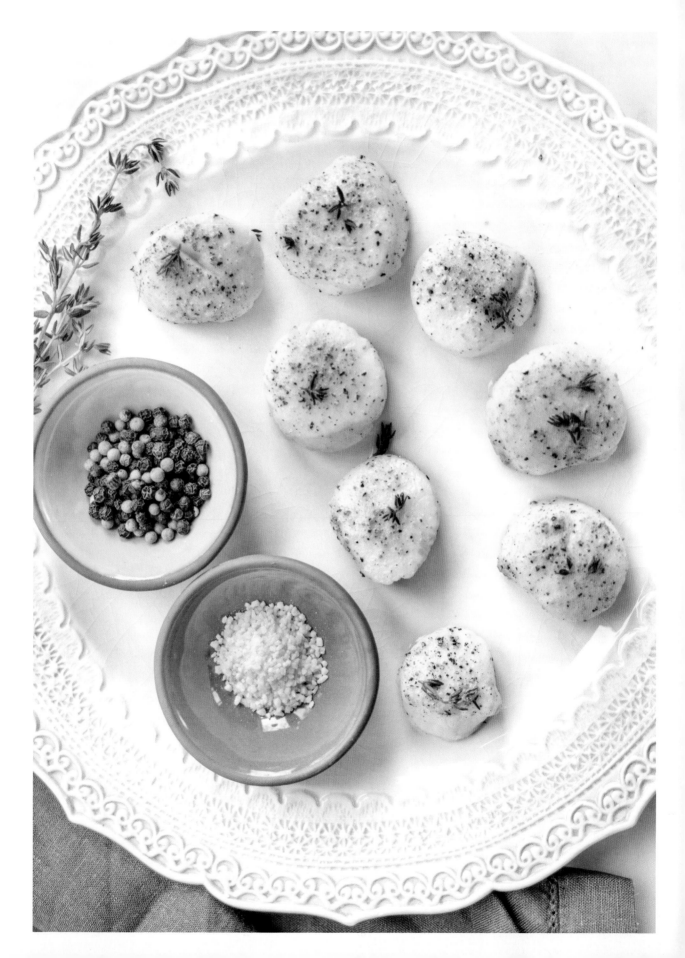

Tuna Melt Croquettes

2 (5-ounce) cans tuna, drained

1 (8-ounce) package cream cheese, softened

½ cup finely shredded cheddar cheese

2 tablespoons diced onions

2 teaspoons prepared yellow mustard

1 large egg

1½ cups pork dust (see page 19) or powdered Parmesan cheese (see page 19)

Fresh dill, for garnish (optional)

FOR SERVING (OPTIONAL):

Cherry tomatoes

Mayonnaise

Prepared yellow mustard

1. Preheat the air fryer to 400°F.

2. Make the patties: In a large bowl, stir together the tuna, cream cheese, cheddar cheese, onions, mustard, and egg until well combined.

3. Place the pork dust in a shallow bowl.

4. Form the tuna mixture into twelve 1½-inch balls. Roll the balls in the pork dust and use your hands to press it into a thick crust around each ball. Flatten the balls into ½-inch-thick patties.

5. Working in batches to avoid overcrowding, place the patties in the air fryer basket, leaving space between them. Cook for 8 minutes, or until golden brown and crispy, flipping halfway through.

6. Garnish the croquettes with fresh dill, if desired, and serve with cherry tomatoes and dollops of mayo and mustard on the side.

7. Store leftovers in an airtight container in the refrigerator for up to 4 days. Reheat in a preheated 400°F air fryer for about 3 minutes, until heated through.

tip: To make the patties easy to form, chill the tuna mixture in the fridge for at least 2 hours or overnight.

(per serving)   calories **528** | fat **36g** | protein **48g** | total carbs **2g** | fiber **0.3g**

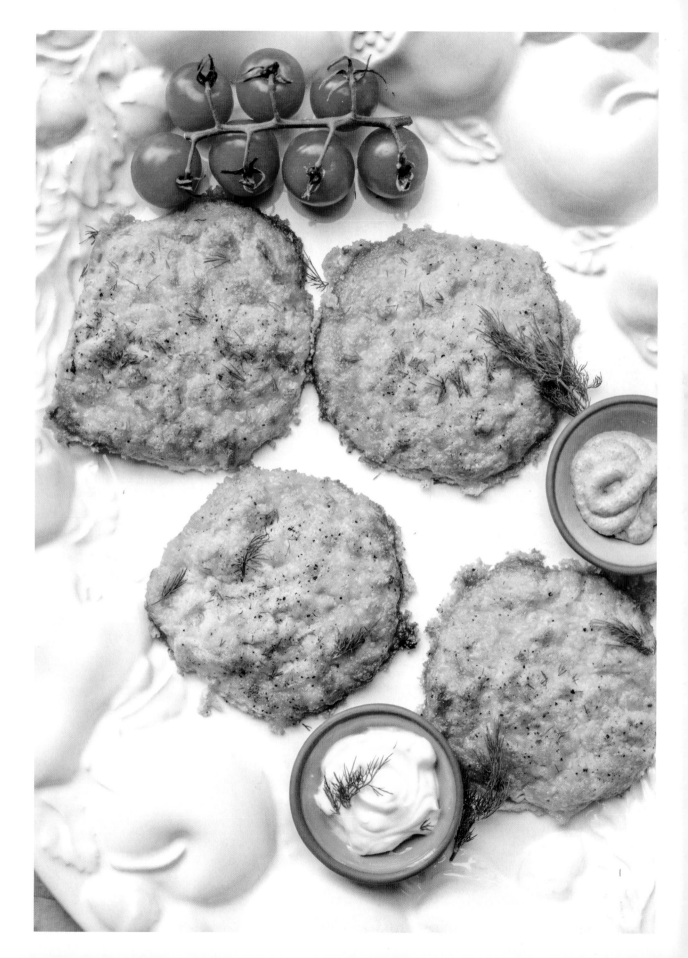

Coconut Shrimp with Spicy Mayo

yield: 4 servings   *prep time:* 10 minutes   *cook time:* 6 minutes

1 pound large shrimp (about 2 dozen), peeled and deveined, tails on

Fine sea salt and ground black pepper

2 large eggs

1 tablespoon water

½ cup unsweetened coconut flakes

½ cup pork dust (see page 19)

SPICY MAYO:

½ cup mayonnaise

2 tablespoons beef or chicken broth

½ teaspoon hot sauce

½ teaspoon cayenne pepper

FOR SERVING (OPTIONAL):

Microgreens

Thinly sliced radishes

1. Spray the air fryer basket with avocado oil. Preheat the air fryer to 400°F.

2. Season the shrimp well on all sides with salt and pepper.

3. Crack the eggs into a shallow baking dish, add the water and a pinch each of salt and pepper, and whisk to combine. In another shallow baking dish, stir together the coconut flakes and pork dust until well combined.

4. Dip one shrimp in the eggs and let any excess egg drip off, then dredge both sides of the shrimp in the coconut mixture. Spray the shrimp with avocado oil and place it in the air fryer basket. Repeat with the remaining shrimp, leaving space between them in the air fryer basket.

5. Cook the shrimp in the air fryer for 6 minutes, or until cooked through and no longer translucent, flipping halfway through.

6. While the shrimp cook, make the spicy mayo: In a medium-sized bowl, stir together all the spicy mayo ingredients until well combined.

7. Serve the shrimp on a bed of microgreens and thinly sliced radishes, if desired. Serve the spicy mayo on the side for dipping.

8. Store leftovers in an airtight container in the refrigerator for up to 4 days. Reheat in a preheated 400°F air fryer for about 3 minutes, until heated through.

(per serving)   calories **360** | fat **28g** | protein **25g** | total carbs **2g** | fiber **1g**

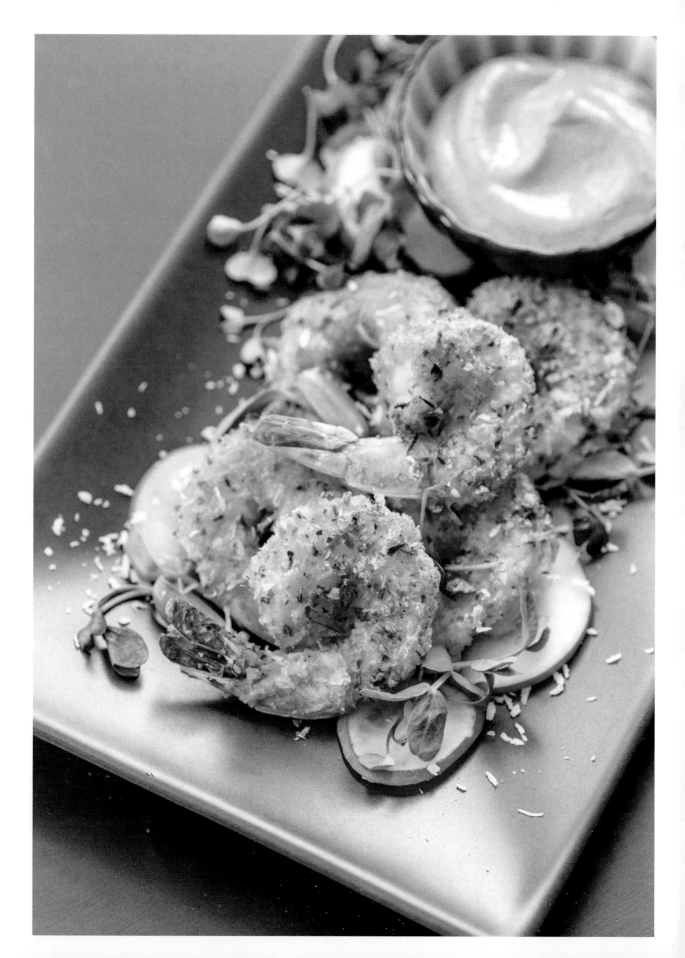

Crispy Crab Rangoon Patties *with Sweet 'n' Sour Sauce*

yield: 8 servings   *prep time:* 10 minutes   *cook time:* 12 minutes per batch

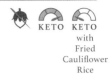

KETO   KETO
with
Fried
Cauliflower
Rice

PATTIES:

1 pound canned lump crabmeat, drained

1 (8-ounce) package cream cheese, softened

1 tablespoon chopped fresh chives

1 large egg

1 teaspoon grated fresh ginger

1 clove garlic, smashed to a paste or minced

COATING:

1½ cups pork dust (see page 19)

DIPPING SAUCE:

½ cup chicken broth

⅓ cup coconut aminos or wheat-free tamari

⅓ cup Swerve confectioners'-style sweetener or equivalent amount of liquid or powdered sweetener (see page 18)

¼ cup tomato sauce

1 tablespoon coconut vinegar or apple cider vinegar

¼ teaspoon grated fresh ginger

1 clove garlic, smashed to a paste

Sliced green onions, for garnish (optional)

Fried Cauliflower Rice (page 98), for serving (optional)

1. Preheat the air fryer to 400°F.

2. In a medium-sized bowl, gently mix all the ingredients for the patties, without breaking up the crabmeat.

3. Form the crab mixture into 8 patties that are 2½ inches in diameter and ¾ inch thick.

4. Place the pork dust in a shallow dish. Place each patty in the pork dust and use your hands to press the pork dust into the patties to form a crust. Place the patties in a single layer in the air fryer, leaving space between them. (If you're using a smaller air fryer, work in batches if necessary.) Cook for 12 minutes, or until the crust is golden and crispy.

5. While the patties cook, make the dipping sauce: In a large saucepan, whisk together all the sauce ingredients. Bring to a simmer over medium-high heat, then turn the heat down to medium until the sauce has reduced and thickened, about 5 minutes. Taste and adjust the seasonings as desired.

6. Place the patties on a serving platter, drizzle with the dipping sauce, and garnish with sliced green onions, if desired. Serve the remaining dipping sauce on the side. Serve with fried cauliflower rice, if desired.

7. Store leftovers in an airtight container in the refrigerator for up to 3 days. Reheat the patties in a preheated 400°F air fryer for 4 minutes, or until crispy on the outside and heated through.

busy family tip: The sauce can be made up to 2 days ahead and stored in an airtight container in the fridge.

(per serving)   calories **411** | fat **30g** | protein **35g** | total carbs **4g** | fiber **3g**

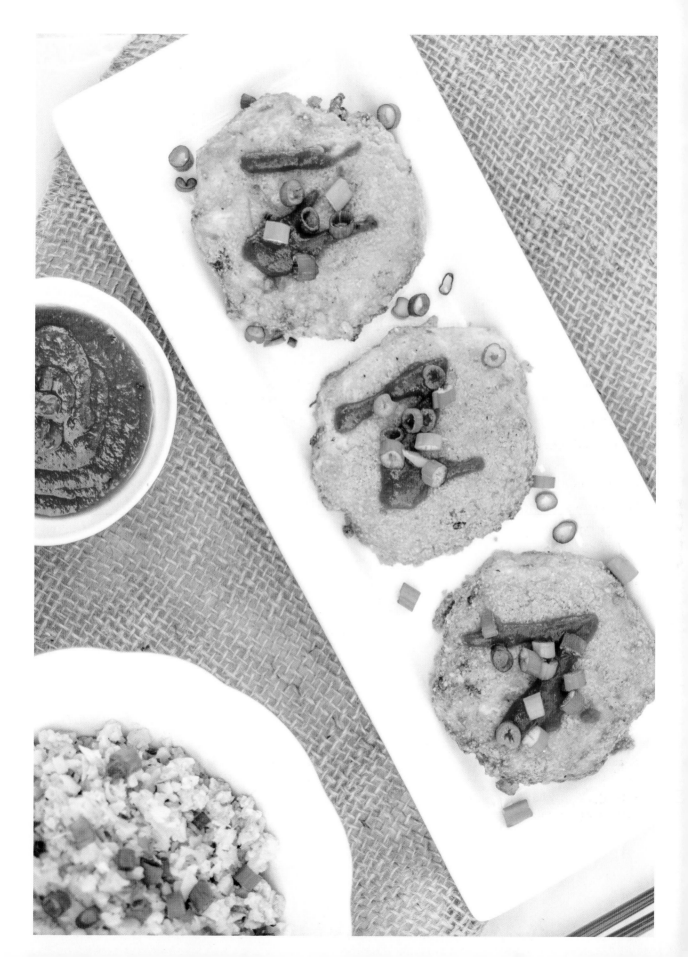

Pecan-Crusted Catfish

yield: 4 servings   *prep time:* 5 minutes   *cook time:* 12 minutes

½ cup pecan meal

1 teaspoon fine sea salt

¼ teaspoon ground black pepper

4 (4-ounce) catfish fillets

FOR GARNISH (OPTIONAL):

Fresh oregano

Pecan halves

1. Spray the air fryer basket with avocado oil. Preheat the air fryer to 375°F.

2. In a large bowl, mix the pecan meal, salt, and pepper. One at a time, dredge the catfish fillets in the mixture, coating them well. Use your hands to press the pecan meal into the fillets. Spray the fish with avocado oil and place them in the air fryer basket.

3. Cook the coated catfish for 12 minutes, or until it flakes easily and is no longer translucent in the center, flipping halfway through.

4. Garnish with oregano sprigs and pecan halves, if desired.

5. Store leftovers in an airtight container in the fridge for up to 3 days. Reheat in a preheated 350°F air fryer for 4 minutes, or until heated through.

(per serving)   calories 162 | fat 11g | protein 17g | total carbs 1g | fiber 1g

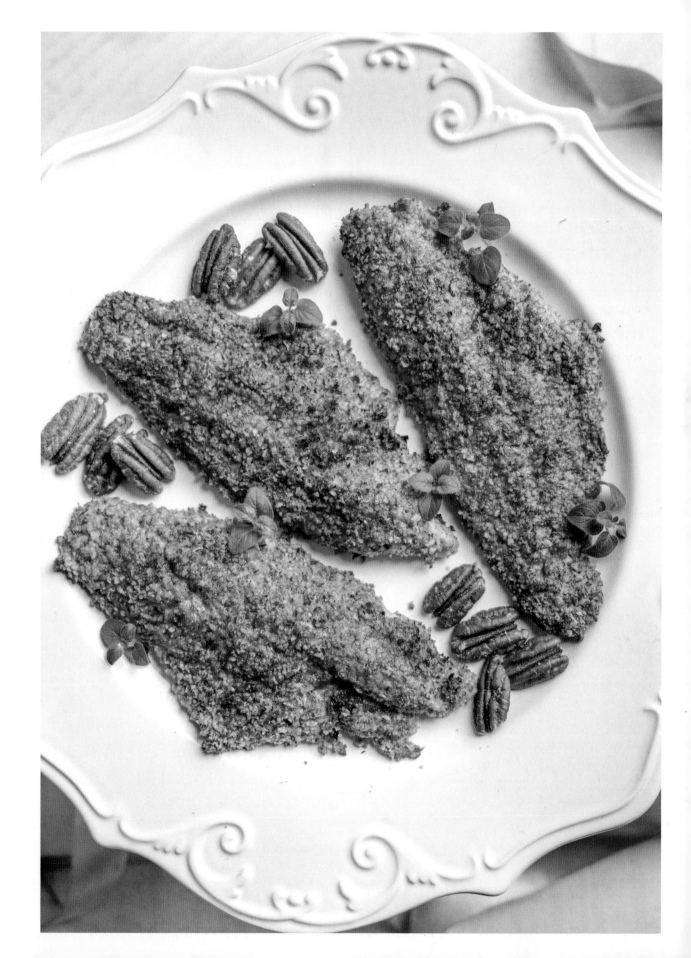

Friday Night Fish Fry

yield: 4 servings *prep time:* 10 minutes *cook time:* 10 minutes

option   KETO

1 large egg

½ cup powdered Parmesan cheese (about 1½ ounces; see page 19) (or pork dust for dairy-free; see page 19)

1 teaspoon smoked paprika

¼ teaspoon celery salt

¼ teaspoon ground black pepper

4 (4-ounce) cod fillets

Chopped fresh oregano or parsley, for garnish (optional)

Lemon slices, for serving (optional)

1. Spray the air fryer basket with avocado oil. Preheat the air fryer to 400°F.

2. Crack the egg in a shallow bowl and beat it lightly with a fork. Combine the Parmesan cheese, paprika, celery salt, and pepper in a separate shallow bowl.

3. One at a time, dip the fillets into the egg, then dredge them in the Parmesan mixture. Using your hands, press the Parmesan onto the fillets to form a nice crust. As you finish, place the fish in the air fryer basket.

4. Cook the fish in the air fryer for 10 minutes, or until it is cooked through and flakes easily with a fork. Garnish with fresh oregano or parsley and serve with lemon slices, if desired.

5. Store leftovers in an airtight container in the refrigerator for up to 3 days. Reheat in a preheated 400°F air fryer for 5 minutes, or until warmed through.

(per serving)   calories **164** | fat **5g** | protein **26g** | total carbs **1g** | fiber **0.2g**

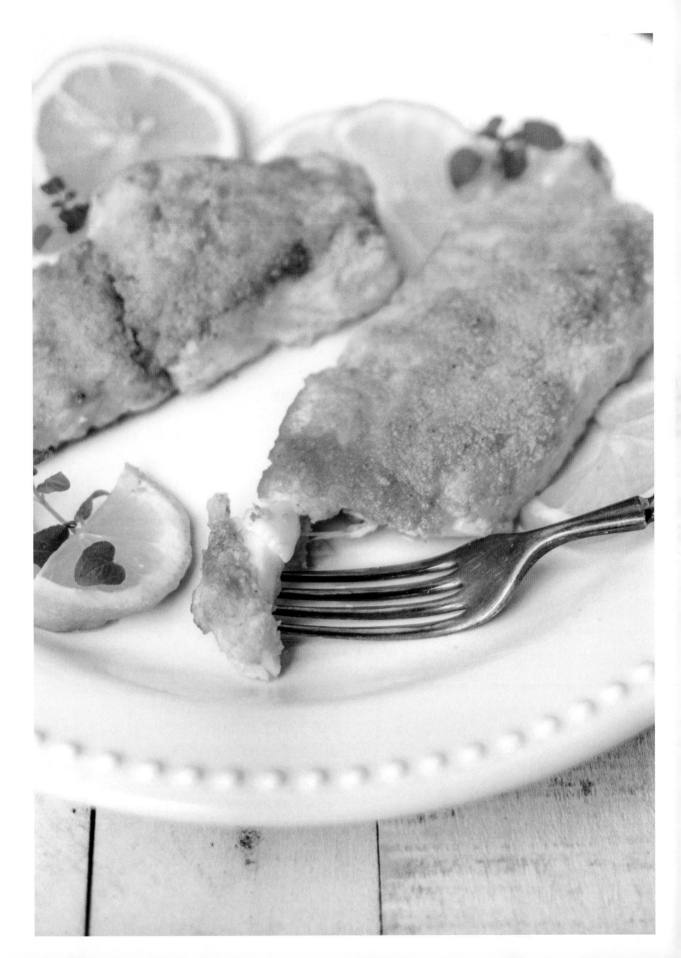

Parmesan-Crusted Shrimp over Pesto Zoodles

yield: 4 servings   *prep time:* 10 minutes   *cook time:* 7 minutes per batch

option   KETO

2 large eggs

3 cloves garlic, minced

2 teaspoons dried basil, divided

½ teaspoon fine sea salt

½ teaspoon ground black pepper

½ cup powdered Parmesan cheese (about 1½ ounces) (see page 19)

1 pound jumbo shrimp, peeled, deveined, butterflied, tails removed

PESTO:

1 packed cup fresh basil

¼ cup extra-virgin olive oil or avocado oil

¼ cup grated Parmesan cheese

¼ cup roasted, salted walnuts (omit for nut-free)

3 cloves garlic, peeled

1 tablespoon lemon juice

½ teaspoon fine sea salt

¼ teaspoon ground black pepper

2 recipes Perfect Zoodles (page 95), warm, for serving

1. Spray the air fryer basket with avocado oil. Preheat the air fryer to 400°F.

2. In a large bowl, whisk together the eggs, garlic, 1 teaspoon of the dried basil, the salt, and the pepper. In a separate small bowl, mix together the remaining teaspoon of dried basil and the Parmesan cheese.

3. Place the shrimp in the bowl with the egg mixture and use your hands to coat the shrimp. Roll one shrimp in the Parmesan mixture and press the coating onto the shrimp with your hands. Place the coated shrimp in the air fryer basket. Repeat with the remaining shrimp, leaving space between them in the air fryer basket. (If you're using a smaller air fryer, work in batches if necessary.)

4. Cook the shrimp in the air fryer for 7 minutes, or until cooked through and no longer translucent, flipping after 4 minutes.

5. While the shrimp cook, make the pesto: Place all the ingredients for the pesto in a food processor and pulse until smooth, with a few rough pieces of basil.

6. Just before serving, toss the warm zoodles with the pesto and place the shrimp on top.

7. Store leftover shrimp and pesto zoodles in separate airtight containers in the refrigerator for up to 3 days or in the freezer for up to a month. Reheat the shrimp in a preheated 400°F air fryer for 5 minutes, or until warmed through. To reheat the pesto zoodles, place them in a casserole dish that will fit in your air fryer and cook at 350°F for 2 minutes, or until heated through.

note: I butterflied the jumbo shrimp in this recipe to reduce the cooking time and create a larger surface area for the crust. To butterfly shrimp, all you have to do is cut from head to tail with a sharp knife and spread the shrimp open.

(per serving)   calories **397** | fat **26g** | protein **31g** | total carbs **10g** | fiber **3g**

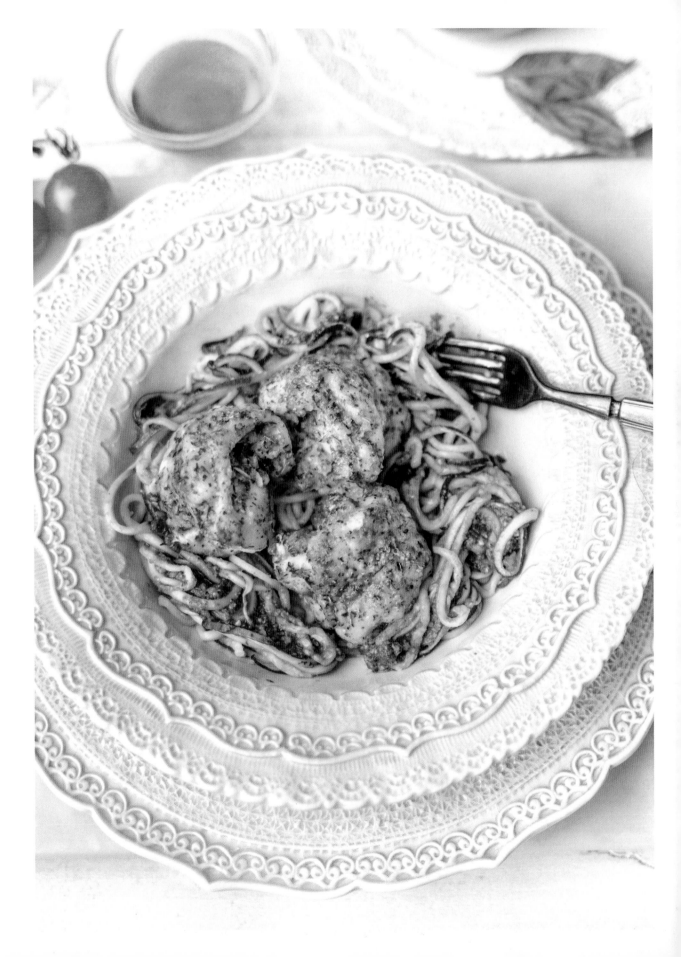

Asian Marinated Salmon

yield: 2 servings *prep time:* 5 minutes, plus 2 hours to marinate *cook time:* 6 minutes

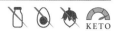

MARINADE:

¼ cup wheat-free tamari or coconut aminos

2 tablespoons lime or lemon juice

2 tablespoons sesame oil

2 tablespoons Swerve confectioners'-style sweetener, or a few drops liquid stevia

2 teaspoons grated fresh ginger

2 cloves garlic, minced

½ teaspoon ground black pepper

2 (4-ounce) salmon fillets (about 1¼ inches thick)

Sliced green onions, for garnish

SAUCE (OPTIONAL):

¼ cup beef broth

¼ cup wheat-free tamari

3 tablespoons Swerve confectioners'-style sweetener or equivalent amount of liquid or powdered sweetener (see page 18)

1 tablespoon tomato sauce

1 teaspoon stevia glycerite (optional)

⅛ teaspoon guar gum or xanthan gum (optional, for thickening)

1. Make the marinade: In a medium-sized shallow dish, stir together all the ingredients for the marinade until well combined. Place the salmon in the marinade. Cover and refrigerate for at least 2 hours or overnight.

2. Preheat the air fryer to 400°F.

3. Remove the salmon fillets from the marinade and place them in the air fryer, leaving space between them. Cook for 6 minutes, or until the salmon is cooked through and flakes easily with a fork.

4. While the salmon cooks, make the sauce, if using: Place all the sauce ingredients except the guar gum in a medium-sized bowl and stir until well combined. Taste and adjust the sweetness to your liking. While whisking slowly, add the guar gum. Allow the sauce to thicken for 3 to 5 minutes. (The sauce can be made up to 3 days ahead and stored in an airtight container in the fridge.) Drizzle the sauce over the salmon before serving.

5. Garnish the salmon with sliced green onions before serving. Store leftovers in an airtight container in the fridge for up to 3 days. Reheat in a preheated 350°F air fryer for 3 minutes, or until heated through.

(per serving) calories **311** | fat **18g** | protein **31g** | total carbs **9g** | fiber **1g**

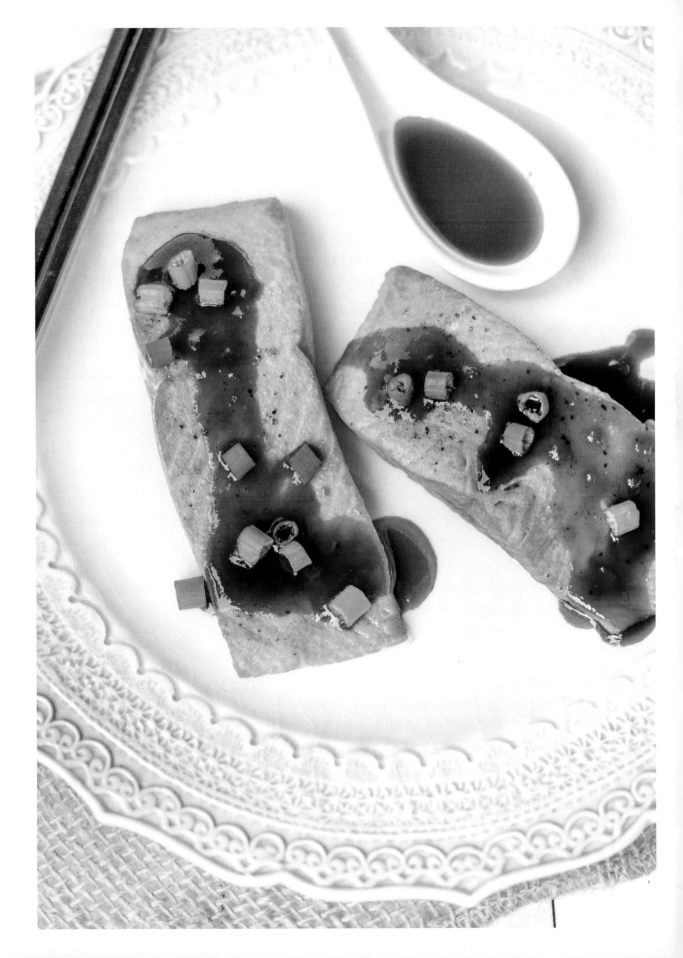

BLT Crab Cakes

yield: 4 servings   *prep time:* 10 minutes   *cook time:* 19 minutes

4 slices bacon

CRAB CAKES:

1 pound canned lump crabmeat, drained well

¼ cup plus 1 tablespoon powdered Parmesan cheese (see page 19) (or pork dust for dairy-free; see page 19)

3 tablespoons mayonnaise

1 large egg

½ teaspoon dried chives

½ teaspoon dried parsley

½ teaspoon dried dill weed

¼ teaspoon garlic powder

¼ teaspoon onion powder

⅛ teaspoon ground black pepper

1 cup pork dust (see page 19)

FOR SERVING:

Leaves from 1 small head Boston lettuce

4 slices tomato

¼ cup mayonnaise

1. Spray the air fryer basket with avocado oil. Preheat the air fryer to 350°F.

2. Place the bacon slices in the air fryer, leaving space between them, and cook for 7 to 9 minutes, until crispy. Remove the bacon and increase the heat to 400°F. Set the bacon aside.

3. Make the crab cakes: Place all the crab cake ingredients except the pork dust in a large bowl and mix together with your hands until well blended. Divide the mixture into 4 equal-sized crab cakes (they should each be about 1 inch thick).

4. Place the pork dust in a small bowl. Dredge the crab cakes in the pork dust to coat them well and use your hands to press the pork dust into the cakes.

5. Place the crab cakes in the air fryer basket, leaving space between them, and cook for 10 minutes, or until crispy on the outside.

6. To serve, place 4 lettuce leaves on a serving platter and top each leaf with a slice of tomato, then a crab cake, then a dollop of mayo, and finally a slice of bacon.

7. Store leftovers in an airtight container in the refrigerator for up to 3 days. Reheat in a preheated 350°F air fryer for 6 minutes, or until heated through.

(per serving)   calories **341** | fat **28g** | protein **22g** | total carbs **3g** | fiber **1g**

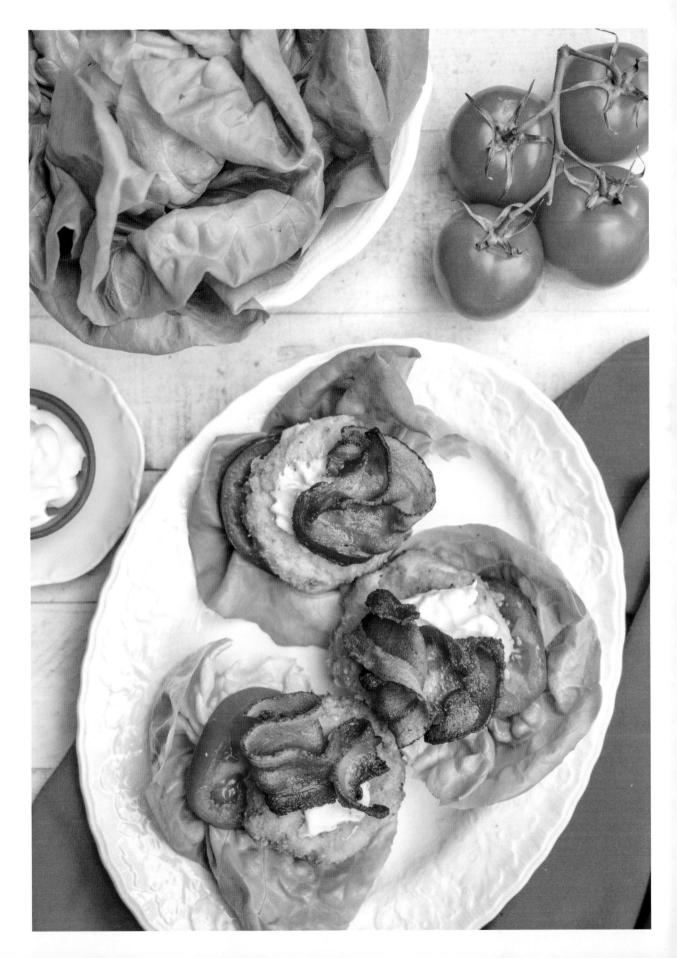

Mouthwatering Cod over Creamy Leek Noodles

yield: 4 servings   *prep time:* 10 minutes   *cook time:* 24 minutes

KETO

1 small leek, sliced into long thin noodles (about 2 cups)

½ cup heavy cream

2 cloves garlic, minced

1 teaspoon fine sea salt, divided

4 (4-ounce) cod fillets (about 1 inch thick) (see Note)

½ teaspoon ground black pepper

COATING:

¼ cup grated Parmesan cheese

2 tablespoons mayonnaise

2 tablespoons unsalted butter, softened

1 tablespoon chopped fresh thyme, or ½ teaspoon dried thyme leaves, plus more for garnish

1. Preheat the air fryer to 350°F.

2. Place the leek noodles in a 6-inch casserole dish or a pan that will fit in your air fryer.

3. In a small bowl, stir together the cream, garlic, and ½ teaspoon of the salt. Pour the mixture over the leeks and cook in the air fryer for 10 minutes, or until the leeks are very tender.

4. Pat the fish dry and season with the remaining ½ teaspoon of salt and the pepper. When the leeks are ready, open the air fryer and place the fish fillets on top of the leeks. Cook for 8 to 10 minutes, until the fish flakes easily with a fork (the thicker the fillets, the longer this will take).

5. While the fish cooks, make the coating: In a small bowl, combine the Parmesan, mayo, butter, and thyme.

6. When the fish is ready, remove it from the air fryer and increase the heat to 425°F (or as high as your air fryer can go). Spread the fillets with a ½-inch-thick to ¾-inch-thick layer of the coating.

7. Place the fish back in the air fryer and cook for 3 to 4 minutes, until the coating browns.

8. Garnish with fresh or dried thyme, if desired. Store leftovers in an airtight container in the refrigerator for up to 3 days. Reheat in a casserole dish in a preheated 350°F air fryer for 6 minutes, or until heated through.

note: While in Maui, I made many variations of this dish using opakapaka and ono in place of the cod. If you have other varieties of fish, feel free to use those instead!

(per serving)   calories **345** | fat **25g** | protein **25g** | total carbs **3g** | fiber **0.4g**

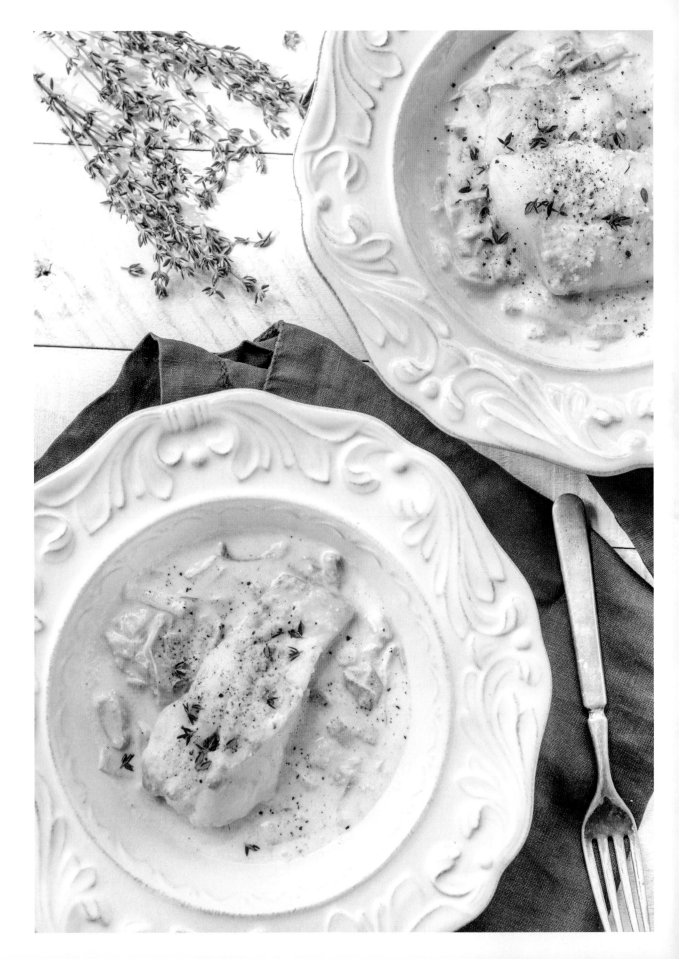

Spicy Popcorn Shrimp

yield: 4 servings *prep time:* 10 minutes *cook time:* 9 minutes

4 large egg yolks

1 teaspoon prepared yellow mustard

1 pound small shrimp, peeled, deveined, and tails removed

½ cup finely shredded Gouda or Parmesan cheese (see Note)

½ cup pork dust (see page 19)

1 tablespoon Cajun seasoning

FOR SERVING/GARNISH (OPTIONAL):

Prepared yellow mustard

Ranch Dressing (page 68)

Tomato sauce

Sprig of fresh parsley

1. Spray the air fryer basket with avocado oil. Preheat the air fryer to 400°F.

2. Place the egg yolks in a large bowl, add the mustard, and whisk until well combined. Add the shrimp and stir well to coat.

3. In a medium-sized bowl, mix together the cheese, pork dust, and Cajun seasoning until well combined.

4. One at a time, roll the coated shrimp in the pork dust mixture and use your hands to press it onto the shrimp. Spray the coated shrimp with avocado oil and place them in the air fryer basket, leaving space between them.

5. Cook the shrimp in the air fryer for 9 minutes, or until cooked through and no longer translucent, flipping after 4 minutes.

6. Serve with your dipping sauces of choice and garnish with a sprig of fresh parsley. Store leftovers in an airtight container in the refrigerator for up to 3 days. Reheat in a preheated 400°F air fryer for 5 minutes, or until warmed through.

note: For this recipe, make sure you use really small pieces of shredded cheese. I pulse shredded cheese in a food processor a few times to break it up into tiny pieces.

(per serving) calories **199** | fat **9g** | protein **27g** | total carbs **1g** | fiber **0g**

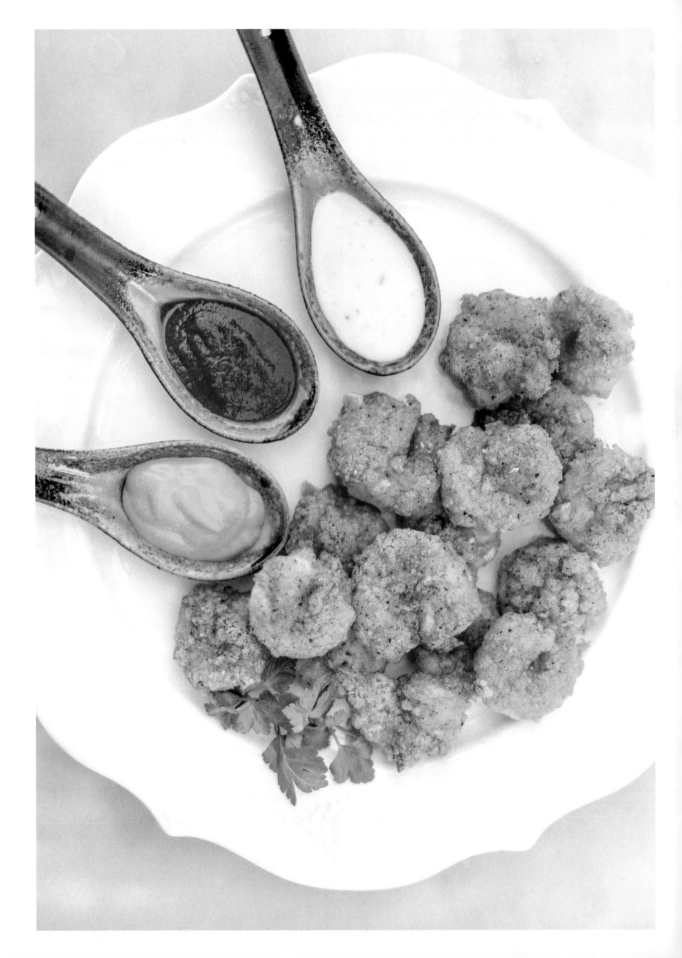

Breaded Shrimp Tacos

yield: 8 tacos (2 per serving) *prep time:* 10 minutes *cook time:* 9 minutes

KETO

2 large eggs

1 teaspoon prepared yellow mustard

1 pound small shrimp, peeled, deveined, and tails removed

½ cup finely shredded Gouda or Parmesan cheese (see Note, page 210)

½ cup pork dust (see page 19)

FOR SERVING:

8 large Boston lettuce leaves

¼ cup pico de gallo

¼ cup shredded purple cabbage

1 lemon, sliced

Guacamole (optional)

1. Preheat the air fryer to 400°F.

2. Crack the eggs into a large bowl, add the mustard, and whisk until well combined. Add the shrimp and stir well to coat.

3. In a medium-sized bowl, mix together the cheese and pork dust until well combined.

4. One at a time, roll the coated shrimp in the pork dust mixture and use your hands to press it onto each shrimp. Spray the coated shrimp with avocado oil and place them in the air fryer basket, leaving space between them.

5. Cook the shrimp for 9 minutes, or until cooked through and no longer translucent, flipping after 4 minutes.

6. To serve, place a lettuce leaf on a serving plate, place several shrimp on top, and top with 1½ teaspoons each of pico de gallo and purple cabbage. Squeeze some lemon juice on top and serve with guacamole, if desired.

7. Store leftover shrimp in an airtight container in the refrigerator for up to 3 days. Reheat in a preheated 400°F air fryer for 5 minutes, or until warmed through.

(per serving) calories **194** | fat **8g** | protein **28g** | total carbs **3g** | fiber **0.5g**

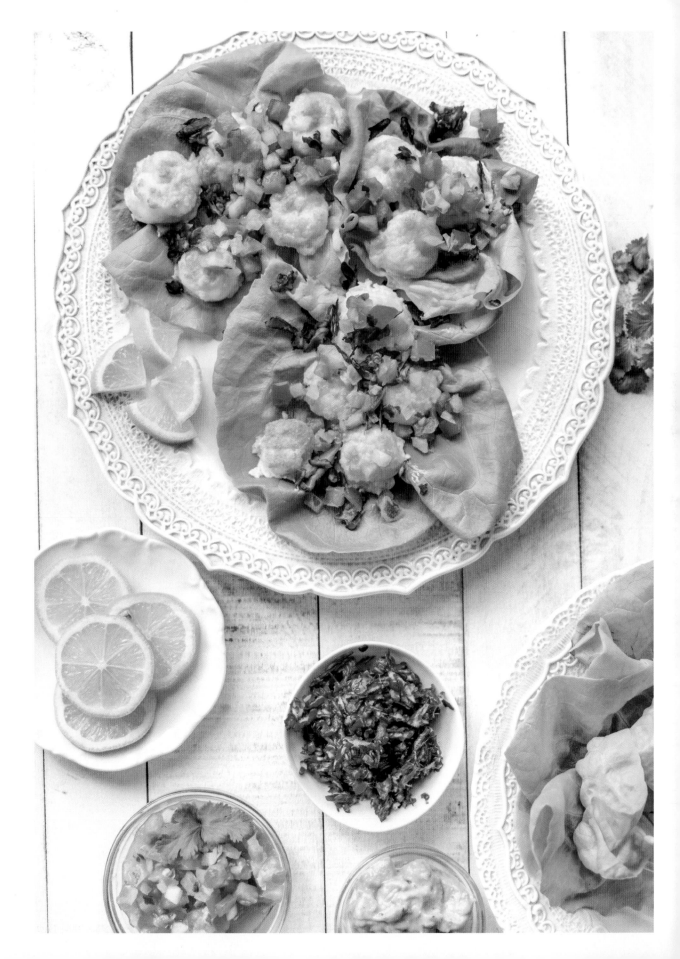

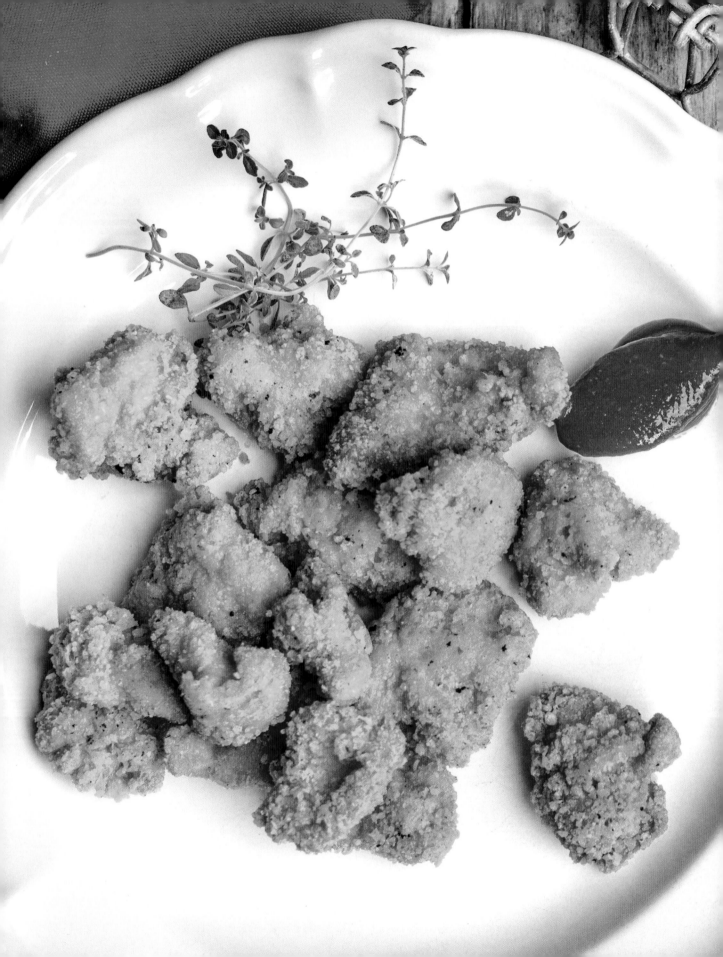

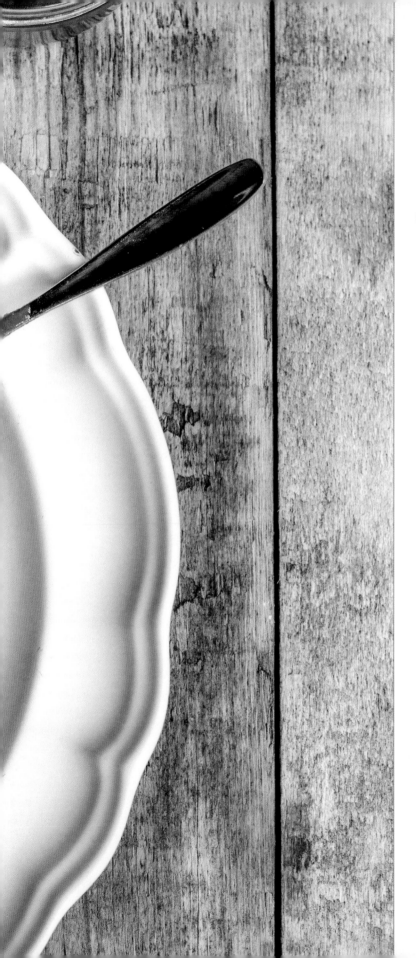

Kid Classics

Ham 'n' Cheese Hand Pies

yield: 4 hand pies (1 per serving)   *prep time:* 10 minutes   *cook time:* 12 minutes

KETO

DOUGH:

1¾ cups shredded mozzarella cheese (about 7 ounces)

2 tablespoons unsalted butter

1 large egg

¾ cup blanched almond flour

⅛ teaspoon fine sea salt

FILLING:

8 thin slices ham

4 slices provolone or cheddar cheese

¼ cup mayonnaise

Prepared yellow mustard, for serving (optional)

busy family tip: These hand pies are super tasty and really cute. If you love them as much as my family does, I highly suggest making a quadruple batch and storing unbaked pies in the freezer for easy meals. Then all you'll have to do for dinner is pop them in the air fryer!

1. Make the dough: Place the mozzarella cheese and butter in a large microwave-safe bowl and microwave for 1 to 2 minutes, until the cheese is entirely melted. Stir well. Add the egg and, using a hand mixer, combine well. Add the almond flour and salt and combine well with the mixer.

2. Lay a piece of parchment paper on the countertop, spray it with avocado oil, and place the dough on it. Knead for about 3 minutes. The dough should be thick yet pliable. (Note: If the dough is too sticky, chill it in the refrigerator for an hour or overnight.)

3. Spray the air fryer basket with avocado oil. Preheat the air fryer to 350°F.

4. Separate the dough into 4 equal portions. Pat each portion out with your hands to form a small circle, about 4 inches in diameter.

5. Place 2 slices of ham and one slice of cheese in the center of each dough circle and smear a tablespoon of mayo on top. Seal each pie closed by folding the dough circle in half and crimping the edges with your fingers.

6. Transfer the pies to the air fryer basket, leaving space between them. Cook for 10 minutes, or until golden brown. Drizzle with mustard before serving, if desired.

7. Store leftovers in an airtight container in the refrigerator for up to 3 days. Reheat in a preheated 350°F air fryer for 3 minutes, or until warmed through.

(per serving)   calories **484** | fat **41g** | protein **26g** | total carbs **6g** | fiber **2g**

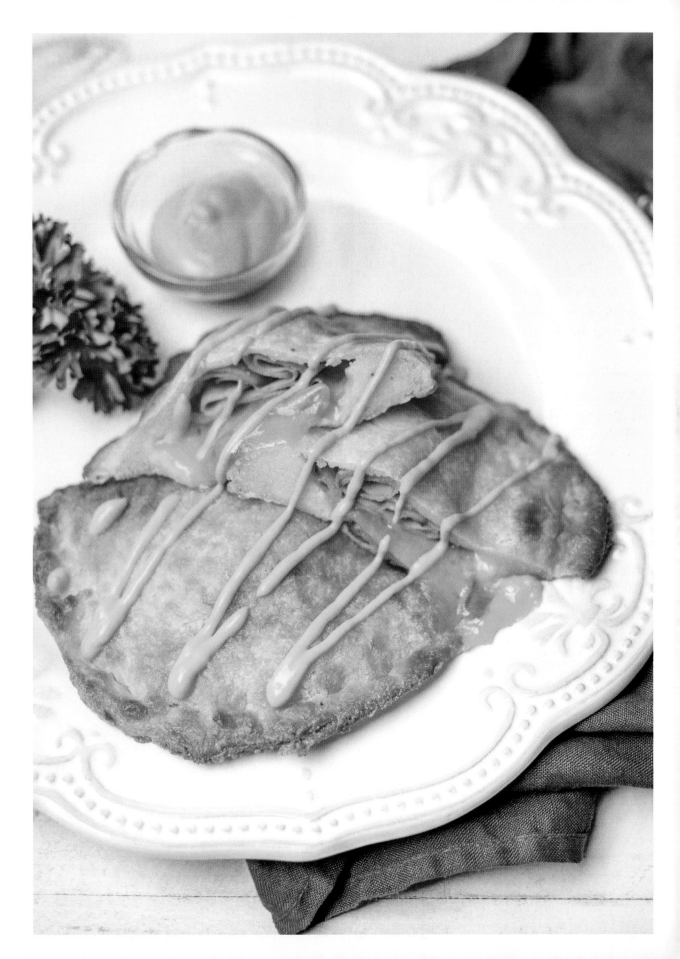

Cheeseburger Meatballs

yield: 4 servings   *prep time:* 10 minutes   *cook time:* 16 minutes

KETO

1 pound ground beef

¼ cup diced onions

1 large egg

1½ teaspoons smoked paprika

½ teaspoon fine sea salt

½ teaspoon garlic powder

½ teaspoon ground black pepper

1 cup mushrooms (about 8 ounces), finely chopped

½ cup tomato sauce

1 dozen (½-inch) cubes cheddar cheese

FOR SERVING (OPTIONAL):

Prepared yellow mustard

Sugar-free or reduced-sugar ketchup

1. Spray the air fryer basket with avocado oil. Preheat the air fryer to 375°F.

2. In a large bowl, mix together the ground beef, onions, egg, paprika, salt, garlic powder, and pepper until well combined. Add the mushrooms and slowly stir in the tomato sauce. The meat mixture should be very moist but still hold its shape when rolled into meatballs.

3. Divide the meat mixture into 12 equal portions. Place 1 cube of cheese in the center of each portion and form the meat around the cheese into a 2-inch meatball. Arrange the meatballs in a single layer in the air fryer basket, leaving space between them.

4. Cook the meatballs for 8 minutes, flip them over, and lower the temperature to 325°F. Cook for another 6 to 8 minutes, until cooked through.

5. Serve with mustard and ketchup, if desired. Store leftovers in an airtight container in the refrigerator for up to 4 days or in the freezer for up to 2 months. Reheat in a preheated 350°F air fryer for about 3 minutes, until heated through.

note: If you don't like mushrooms, don't worry—you won't even know they are there! But they add umami, that fifth taste on your tongue (along with salt, sour, bitter, and sweet) that's savory and delicious. Mushrooms also add moisture.

(per serving)   calories **621** | fat **47g** | protein **45g** | total carbs **5g** | fiber **1g**

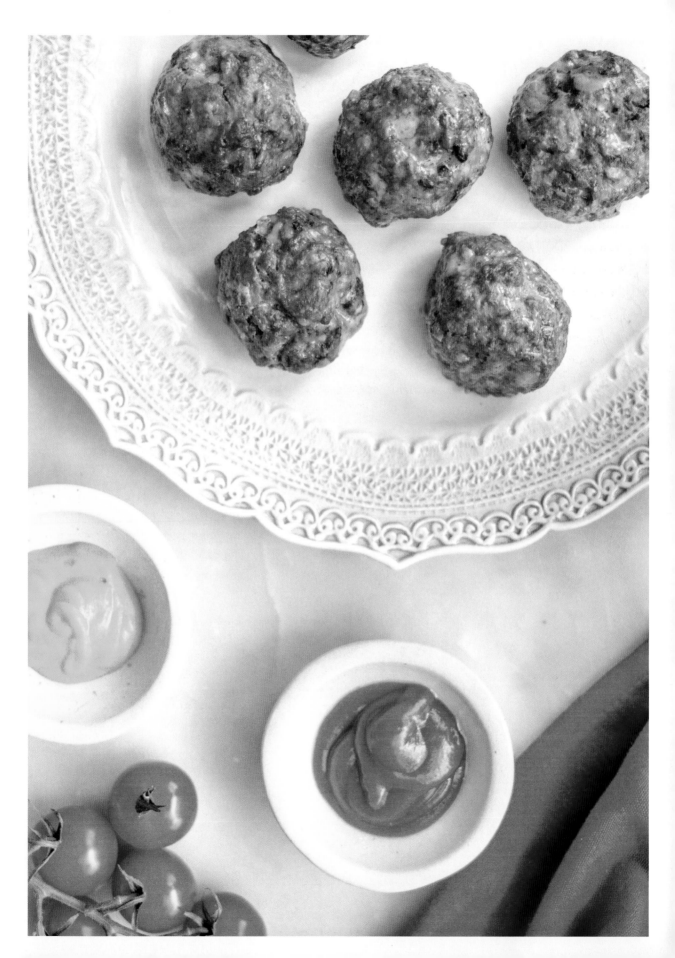

Keto Turtles

yield: 4 servings   *prep time:* 15 minutes   *cook time:* 15 minutes per batch

1 pound ground beef

1 teaspoon fine sea salt

½ teaspoon ground black pepper

4 hot dogs

8 whole peppercorns

2 large dill pickles

2 slices bacon

FOR SERVING:

Prepared yellow mustard

Cornichons

1. Spray the air fryer basket with avocado oil. Preheat the air fryer to 390°F.

2. Create the turtle shells: Form the ground beef into 4 equal-sized patties. Season the outsides of the patties with the salt and pepper.

3. Make the turtle heads: Slice 1½ inches off one end of each hot dog. Use your thumb to make an indent in the side of each ground beef patty and press in a hot dog end for the head. Use the tip of a sharp knife to score 2 spots in each hot dog end for the eyes. Place a whole peppercorn in each slot.

4. Make the turtle legs: Cut the rest of the hot dogs in half lengthwise, then cut each half in half crosswise (you should have sixteen 1½-inch pieces). Place one piece flat side down under each front corner of the patties. (You will have 8 hot dog pieces left over.)

5. Decorate the shells: Cut the dill pickles into ⅛-inch-thick slices that are about 3 inches long. Place the pickle slices parallel to each other on top of the ground beef patties, spaced about half an inch apart.

6. Slice the bacon into ¼-inch-wide and 5- to 6-inch-long strips. Place the strips on the patties, on top of and perpendicular to the pickle slices, spaced about half an inch apart. Tuck the ends of the bacon strips underneath the turtle so they don't curl up.

7. Place the turtles in the air fryer basket, leaving space between them (if you're using a smaller air fryer, work in batches if necessary). Cook for 10 to 15 minutes, until the beef is cooked to your liking.

8. Remove from the air fryer and serve with mustard and cornichons. Store leftovers in an airtight container in the refrigerator for up to 4 days or in the freezer for up to 2 months. Reheat in a preheated 390°F air fryer for about 5 minutes, until heated through.

(per serving)   calories **389** | fat **28g** | protein **30g** | total carbs **0.4g** | fiber **0.1g**

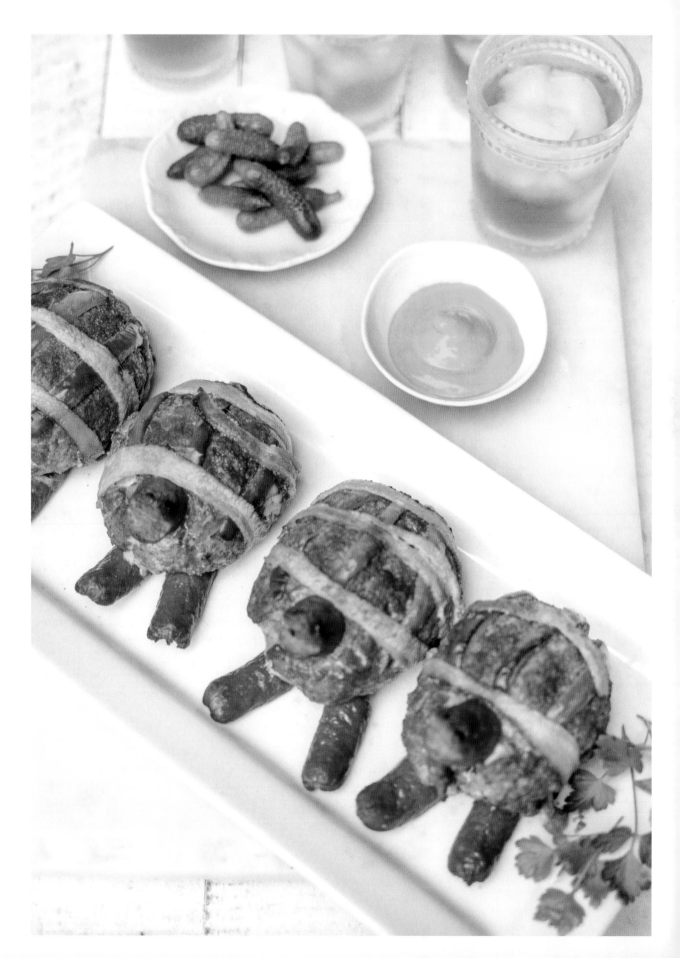

No-Corn Dogs

yield: 4 servings   *prep time*: 10 minutes   *cook time*: 10 minutes

KETO

1¾ cups shredded mozzarella cheese (about 7 ounces)

2 tablespoons unsalted butter

1 large egg

¾ cup blanched almond flour

⅛ teaspoon fine sea salt

4 hot dogs

FOR SERVING (OPTIONAL):

Prepared yellow mustard

No-sugar or reduced-sugar ketchup

busy family tip: *These are such a hit with my little boys that I make a quadruple batch and store the unbaked extras in the freezer. For an easy lunch, all I have to do is thaw two dogs for 20 minutes and heat them in the air fryer for 5 minutes!*

1. Make the dough: Place the mozzarella cheese and butter in a large microwave-safe bowl and microwave for 1 to 2 minutes, until the cheese is entirely melted. Stir well. Add the egg and, using a hand mixer, combine well. Add the almond flour and salt and combine well with the mixer.

2. Lay a piece of parchment paper on the countertop, spray it with avocado oil, and place the dough on it. Knead for about 3 minutes. The dough should be thick yet pliable. (Note: If the dough is too sticky, chill it in the refrigerator for an hour or overnight.)

3. Spray the air fryer basket with avocado oil. Preheat the air fryer to 390°F.

4. Separate the dough into 4 equal portions. Pat each portion out with your hands to form a small oval, about 6 inches long and 2 inches wide.

5. Place one hot dog in each oval and form the dough around each hot dog using your hands. Place the dogs in the air fryer basket, leaving space between them, and cook for 8 minutes, or until golden brown, flipping halfway through. Drizzle with yellow mustard and serve with ketchup on the side, if desired.

6. Store leftovers in an airtight container in the refrigerator for up to 3 days. Reheat in a preheated 350°F air fryer for 5 minutes, or until warmed through.

(per serving)   calories **405** | fat **33g** | protein **24g** | total carbs **5g** | fiber **2g**

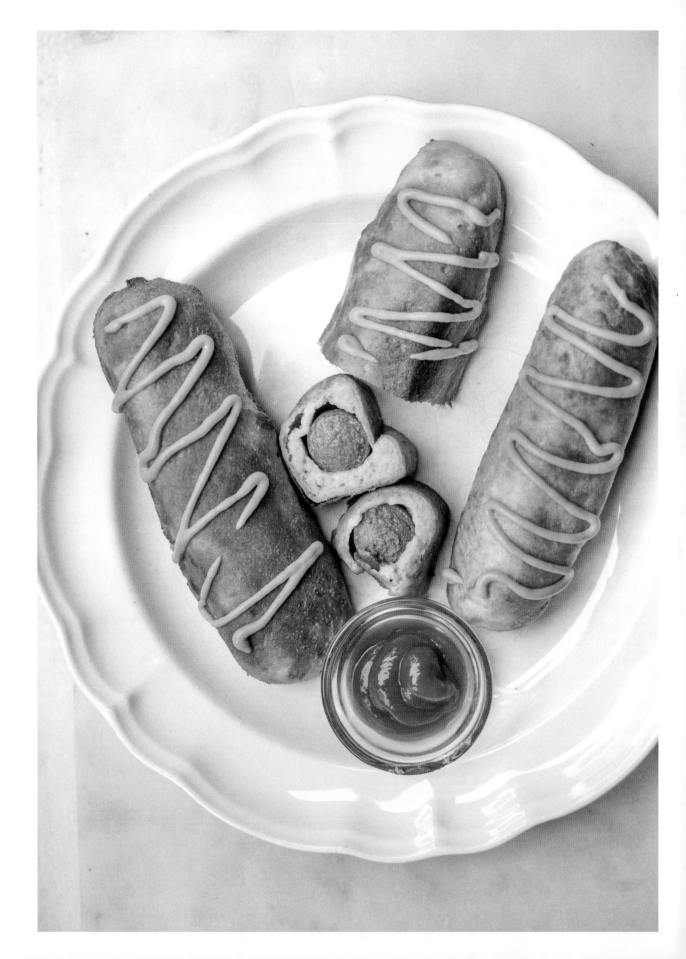

Italian Dunkers

yield: 6 servings   *prep time:* 10 minutes   *cook time:* 8 minutes

2 large eggs

1 cup pork dust (see page 19)

2 teaspoons Italian seasoning

1 pound boneless, skinless chicken tenders

½ cup marinara sauce, for serving

1. Spray the air fryer basket with avocado oil. Preheat the air fryer to 390°F.

2. In a medium-sized bowl, lightly beat the eggs. In another medium-sized bowl, combine the pork dust and Italian seasoning.

3. One at a time, dip the chicken tenders in the eggs, shake off the excess egg, then dredge the tenders in the pork dust mixture. Using your hands, press the coating into each tender, coating it well. Place the tenders in the air fryer basket, leaving space between them.

4. Cook the tenders for 8 minutes, or until the internal temperature reaches 165°F and they are golden brown, flipping halfway through. Transfer the chicken tenders to a platter and serve with the marinara sauce.

5. Store leftovers in an airtight container in the refrigerator for up to 4 days. Reheat in a preheated 390°F air fryer for about 3 minutes, until heated through.

(per serving)   calories **332** | fat **22g** | protein **36g** | total carbs **1g** | fiber **0.3g**

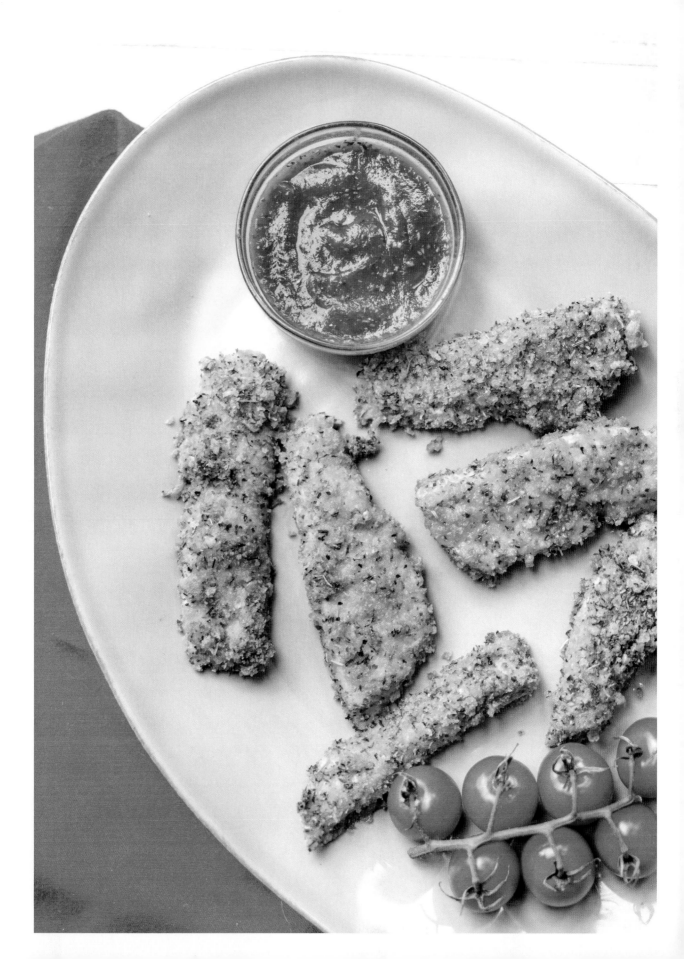

Hot Dog Buns

1½ cups blanched almond flour

¼ cup plus 1 tablespoon psyllium husk powder (see Note)

2 teaspoons baking powder

1 teaspoon fine sea salt

2½ tablespoons apple cider vinegar

3 large egg whites

1 cup boiling water

note: The psyllium husk powder is a must for this recipe—no substitutes! Make sure you purchase a fine powder. And if your buns are purple, don't worry— some brands of psyllium husk powder cause this.

tips: Hot dogs cook perfectly in an air fryer. Preheat the air fryer to 400°F, place 2 hot dogs directly in the air fryer basket, leaving space between them, and cook for 8 minutes, or until crispy on the outside, flipping halfway through.

1. Spray a 7-inch pie pan or a casserole dish that will fit inside your air fryer with avocado oil. Preheat the air fryer to 325°F.

2. In a medium-sized bowl, mix together the flour, psyllium husk powder, baking powder, and salt until well combined. Add the vinegar and egg whites and stir until a thick dough forms. Add the boiling water and mix until well combined. Let sit for 1 to 2 minutes, until the dough firms up.

3. Divide the dough into 8 equal-sized balls. Form each ball into a hot dog shape that's about 1 inch wide and 3½ inches long. Place the buns in the greased pie pan, spacing them about 1 inch apart.

4. Place the buns in the air fryer and cook for 15 minutes, then flip the buns over. Cook for another 5 to 10 minutes, until the buns are puffed up and cooked through and a toothpick inserted in the center of a bun comes out clean.

5. Store leftovers in an airtight container in the fridge for up to 5 days or in the freezer for up to a month.

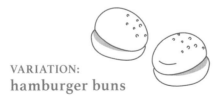

VARIATION:
hamburger buns

To make burger buns, shape the dough into 2½-inch balls and place them in the greased pie pan 2 inches apart. Bake as instructed in step 4.

(per serving)   calories **145** | fat **11g** | protein **6g** | total carbs **10g** | fiber **7g**

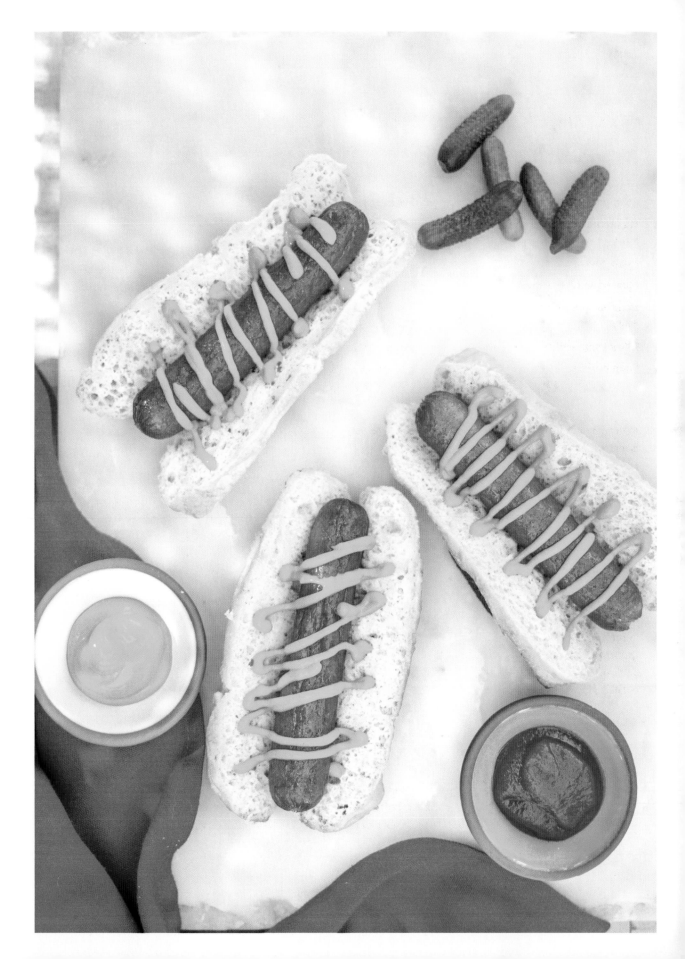

BLT Sushi

yield: 4 servings   *prep time:* 15 minutes   *cook time:* 8 minutes

8 slices thin-cut bacon

¼ cup mayonnaise

1½ cups shredded lettuce

1 cup diced tomatoes

1. Preheat the air fryer to 400°F.

2. Remove the air fryer basket from the air fryer and place the bacon in it. Weave the bacon slices together in a square, 4 slices per side, threading each slice over and under the others. Make sure the grid is tight; if there are gaps, the mayo will leak through.

3. Return the air fryer basket to the air fryer and cook the bacon for 8 minutes, or until slightly crisp yet still flexible.

4. Place the bacon square on a cutting board crispy side down. Spread the mayo over the bacon. Place the shredded lettuce and tomatoes on the mayo. Roll the bacon square up tightly. Slice into 4 thick rolls and serve.

5. Best served fresh. Store leftovers in an airtight container in the fridge for up to 4 days. Serve leftovers chilled or reheat in a preheated 400°F air fryer for 5 minutes, or until heated through.

tip: *If you have a small round air fryer and the woven bacon square doesn't fit, you can also bake it in the oven for the same amount of time.*

(per serving)   calories **254** | fat **22g** | protein **9g** | total carbs **5g** | fiber **2g**

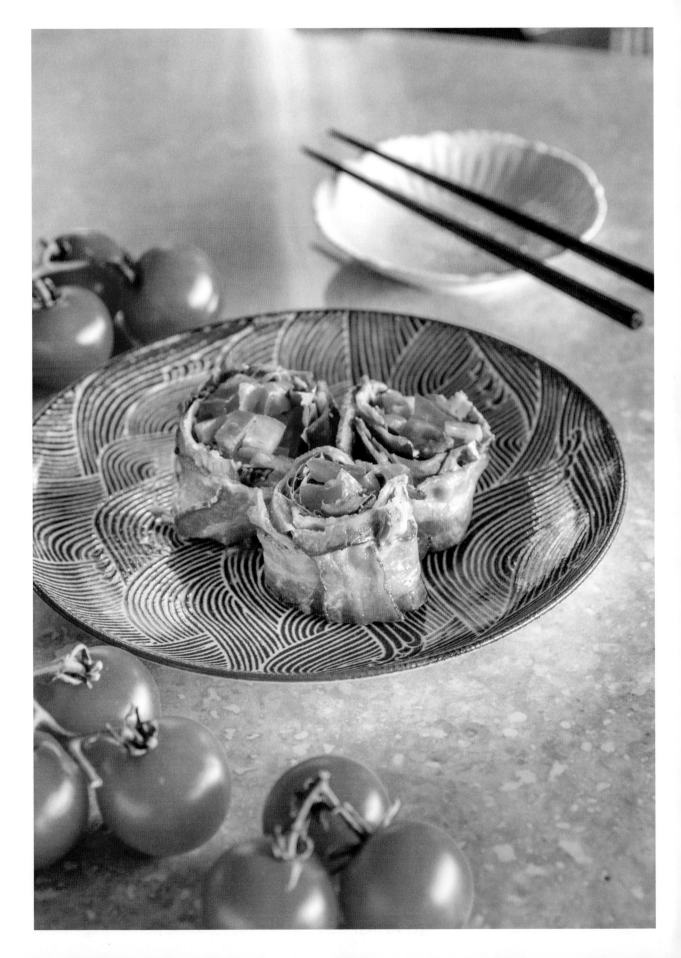

Popcorn Chicken

yield: 4 servings   *prep time:* 10 minutes   *cook time:* 15 minutes

KETO

½ cup mayonnaise

1 teaspoon prepared yellow mustard

½ cup finely shredded cheddar cheese (about 2 ounces) (see Note, page 210)

½ cup pork dust (see page 19)

¼ teaspoon garlic powder

¼ teaspoon onion powder

¼ teaspoon smoked paprika

1 pound boneless, skinless chicken breasts, cut into ½-inch pieces

Chopped fresh parsley, for garnish (optional)

Ranch Dressing (page 68), for serving (optional)

1. Spray the air fryer basket with avocado oil. Preheat the air fryer to 400°F.

2. In a large bowl, mix together the mayonnaise and mustard. In a separate medium-sized bowl, mix together the cheese, pork dust, garlic powder, onion powder, and paprika until well combined.

3. Add the chicken pieces to the mayonnaise mixture and stir well to coat. One at a time, roll the coated chicken pieces in the pork dust mixture and spray them with avocado oil, then place them in the air fryer basket, leaving space between them.

4. Cook the chicken for 12 to 15 minutes, until the internal temperature reaches 165°F and the coating is golden brown.

5. Garnish with fresh parsley, if desired, and serve with ranch dressing, if desired. Store leftovers in an airtight container in the fridge for up to 4 days. Serve leftovers chilled or reheat in a preheated 400°F air fryer for 5 minutes, or until heated through.

(per serving)   calories **479** | fat **36g** | protein **37g** | total carbs **1g** | fiber **0.1g**

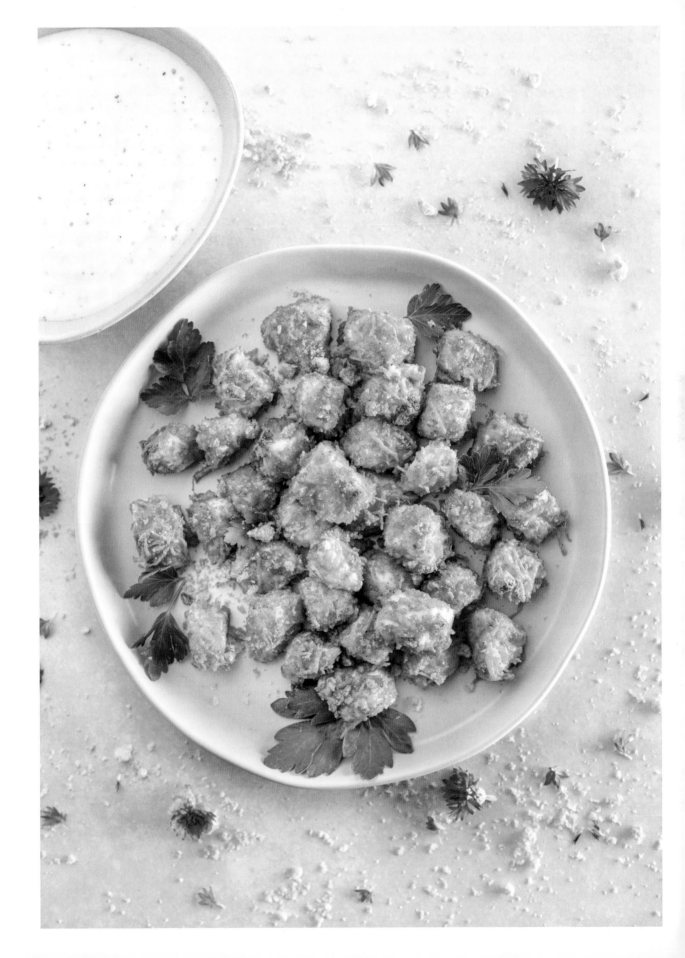

Ham 'n' Cheese Ravioli

yield: 6 servings   *prep time:* 15 minutes   *cook time:* 10 minutes

KETO

1 cup shredded cheddar cheese (about 4 ounces)

6 ounces cream cheese (¾ cup), softened

8 ounces thinly sliced ham (12 very large slices)

1 large egg

1 cup pork dust (see page 19)

Fresh parsley leaves, for garnish (optional)

Ranch Dressing (page 68), for serving (optional)

1. Spray the air fryer basket with avocado oil. Preheat the air fryer to 400°F.

2. In a small bowl, stir together the cheddar cheese and cream cheese until well combined.

3. Assemble the ravioli: Lay one slice of ham on a sheet of parchment paper. Spoon about 2 heaping tablespoons of the filling into the center of the ham. Fold one end of the ham over the filling, making sure the ham completely covers the filling and meets the ham on the other side (otherwise, the filling will leak out). Fold the ends around the filling to make a square, making sure that the filling is covered well. Using your fingers, press down around the filling to even the ravioli out into a square shape. Repeat with the rest of the ham and filling; you should have 12 ravioli.

4. Crack the egg into a shallow bowl and beat well with a fork. Place the pork dust in another shallow bowl.

5. Gently dip each ravioli into the egg, then dredge it in the pork dust. Use your hands to press the pork dust into the ravioli, coating it well. Spray the ravioli with avocado oil and place it in the air fryer basket. Make sure to leave space between the ravioli.

6. Cook the ravioli in the air fryer for 10 minutes, or until crispy, flipping after 6 minutes.

7. Serve warm, garnished with fresh parsley and with ranch dressing for dipping if desired.

8. Store leftovers in an airtight container in the fridge for up to 4 days. Reheat in a preheated 400°F air fryer for 3 minutes, or until heated through.

(per serving)   calories **269** | fat **20g** | protein **16g** | total carbs **4g** | fiber **0.3g**

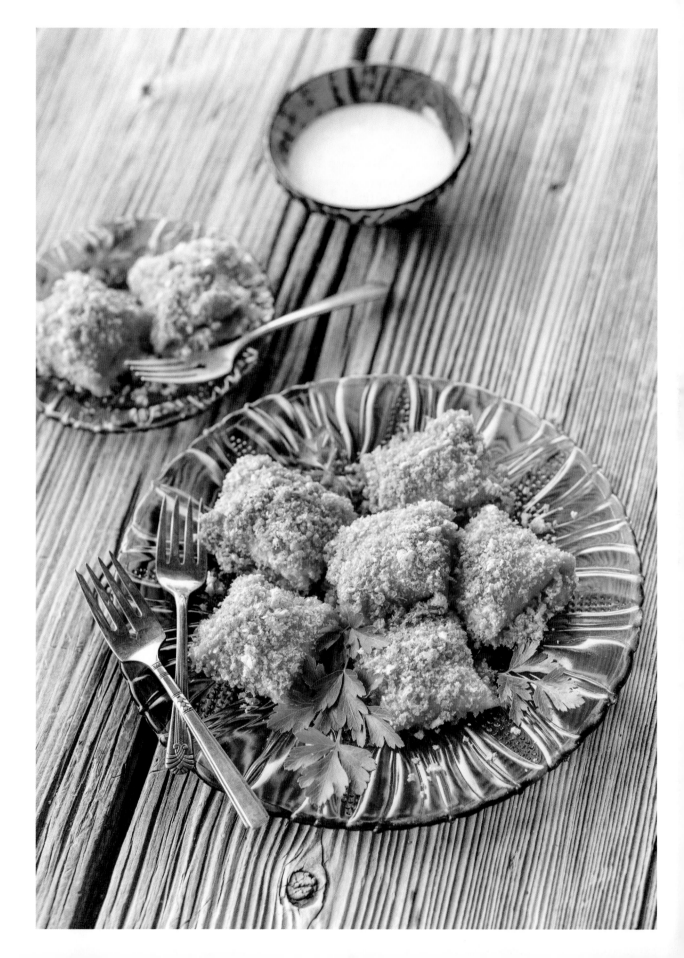

Chicken Patties

yield: 6 servings   *prep time:* 10 minutes   *cook time:* 10 minutes per batch

PATTIES:

1 pound ground chicken

⅓ cup shredded cheddar cheese (omit for dairy-free)

2 tablespoons diced onions, or ¼ teaspoon onion powder

2 tablespoons mayonnaise

1 teaspoon dill pickle juice

1 teaspoon fine sea salt

COATING:

1 cup pork dust (see page 19)

FOR SERVING (OPTIONAL):

Cornichons

Mayonnaise

Prepared yellow mustard

1. Spray the air fryer basket with avocado oil. Preheat the air fryer to 375°F.

2. Place the ingredients for the patties in a medium-sized bowl and use your hands to combine well. Form the mixture into six 3½-inch patties.

3. Place the pork dust in a shallow bowl. Dredge each patty in the pork dust and use your hands to press the pork dust into a crust around the patty.

4. Working in batches if necessary, place the patties in the air fryer basket, leaving space between them, and cook for 5 minutes. Flip the patties with a spatula and cook for another 5 minutes, or until the coating is golden brown and the chicken is no longer pink inside.

5. Serve the patties with cornichons, mayo, and mustard, if desired.

6. Store leftovers in an airtight container in the refrigerator for up to 3 days. Reheat in a preheated 350°F air fryer for 4 minutes, or until heated through.

     (per serving)   calories **352** | fat **25g** | protein **28g** | total carbs **4g** | fiber **3g**

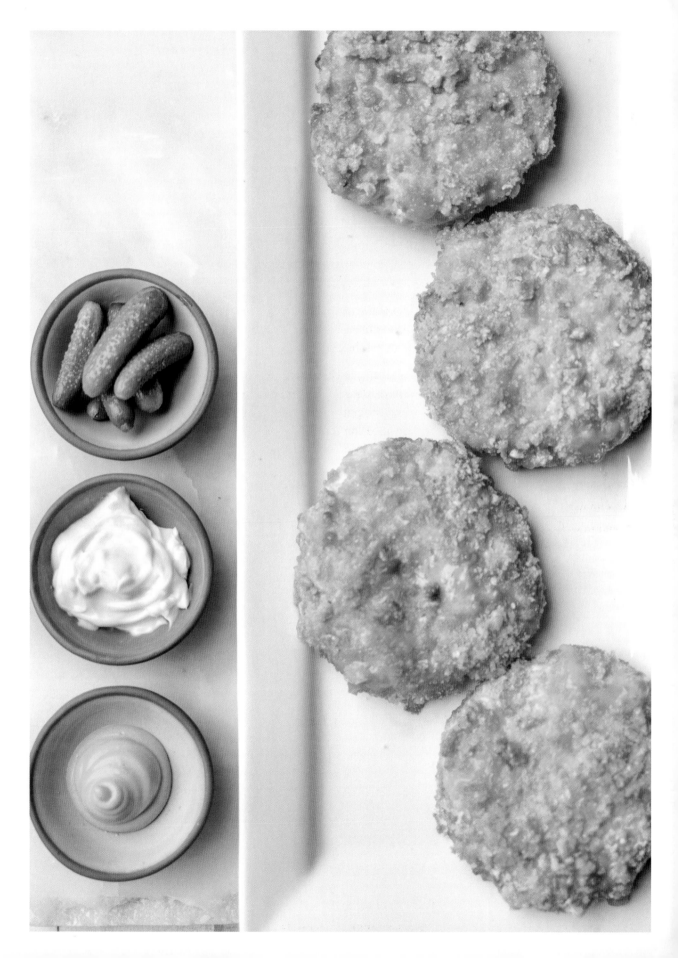

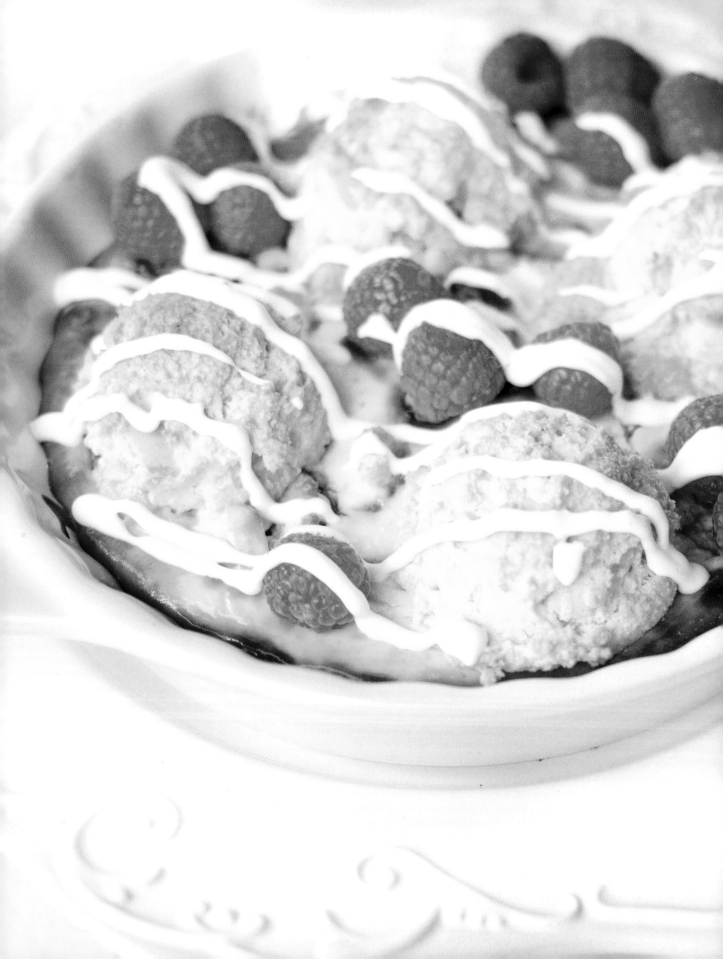

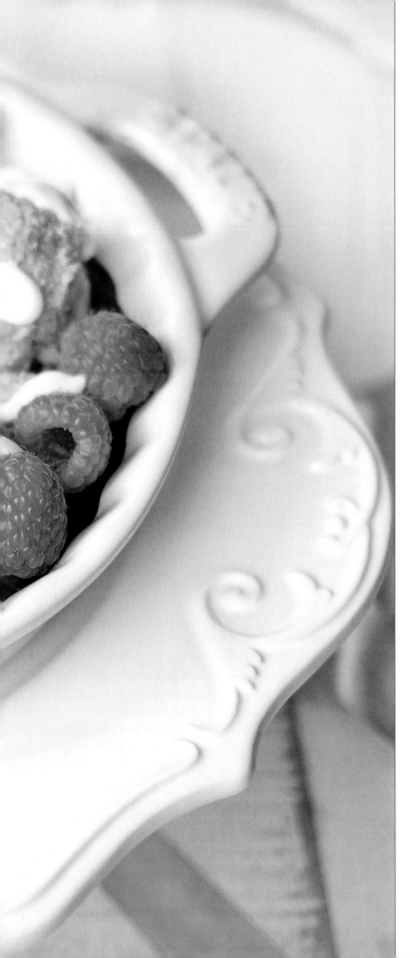

Sweet Endings

Little French Fudge Cakes

yield: 12 cakes (1 per serving) *prep time:* 10 minutes *cook time:* 25 minutes

CAKES:

3 cups blanched almond flour

¾ cup unsweetened cocoa powder

1 teaspoon baking soda

½ teaspoon fine sea salt

6 large eggs

1 cup Swerve confectioners'-style sweetener or equivalent amount of powdered sweetener (see page 18)

1½ cups canned pumpkin puree

3 tablespoons brewed decaf espresso or other strong brewed decaf coffee

3 tablespoons unsalted butter, melted but not hot (or coconut oil for dairy-free)

1 teaspoon vanilla extract

CREAM CHEESE FROSTING:

½ cup Swerve confectioners'-style sweetener or equivalent amount of powdered or liquid sweetener (see page 18)

½ cup (1 stick) unsalted butter, melted (or coconut oil for dairy-free)

4 ounces cream cheese (½ cup) (or Kite Hill brand cream cheese style spread for dairy-free), softened

3 tablespoons unsweetened, unflavored almond milk or heavy cream

CHOCOLATE DRIZZLE:

3 tablespoons unsalted butter, melted (or coconut oil for dairy-free)

2 tablespoons Swerve confectioners'-style sweetener or equivalent amount of powdered or liquid sweetener (see page 18)

2 tablespoons unsweetened cocoa powder

¼ cup unsweetened, unflavored almond milk

+

½ cup chopped walnuts or pecans, for garnish (optional)

1. Preheat the air fryer to 350°F. Spray 2 mini Bundt pans with coconut oil.

2. In a medium-sized bowl, whisk together the flour, cocoa powder, baking soda, and salt until blended.

3. In a large bowl, beat the eggs and sweetener with a hand mixer for 2 to 3 minutes, until light and fluffy. Add the pumpkin puree, espresso, melted butter, and vanilla and stir to combine.

4. Add the wet ingredients to the dry ingredients and stir until just combined.

5. Pour the batter into the prepared pans, filling each well two-thirds full. Cook in the air fryer for 20 to 25 minutes, until a toothpick inserted into the center of a cake comes out clean. Allow the cakes to cool completely in the pans before removing them.

6. Make the frosting: In a large bowl, mix the sweetener, melted butter, and cream cheese until well combined. Add the almond milk and stir well to combine.

7. Make the chocolate drizzle: In a small bowl, stir together the melted butter, sweetener, and cocoa powder until well combined. Add the almond milk while stirring to thin the mixture.

8. After the cakes have cooled, dip the tops of the cakes into the frosting, then use a spoon to drizzle the chocolate over each frosted cake. If desired, garnish the cakes with chopped nuts.

9. Store leftovers in an airtight container in the refrigerator for up to 4 days or in the freezer for up to a month.

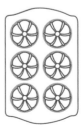

special equipment:

2 (6-well) mini Bundt cake pans (see Tip)

(per serving) calories **414** | fat **38g** | protein **12g** | total carbs **11g** | fiber **5g**

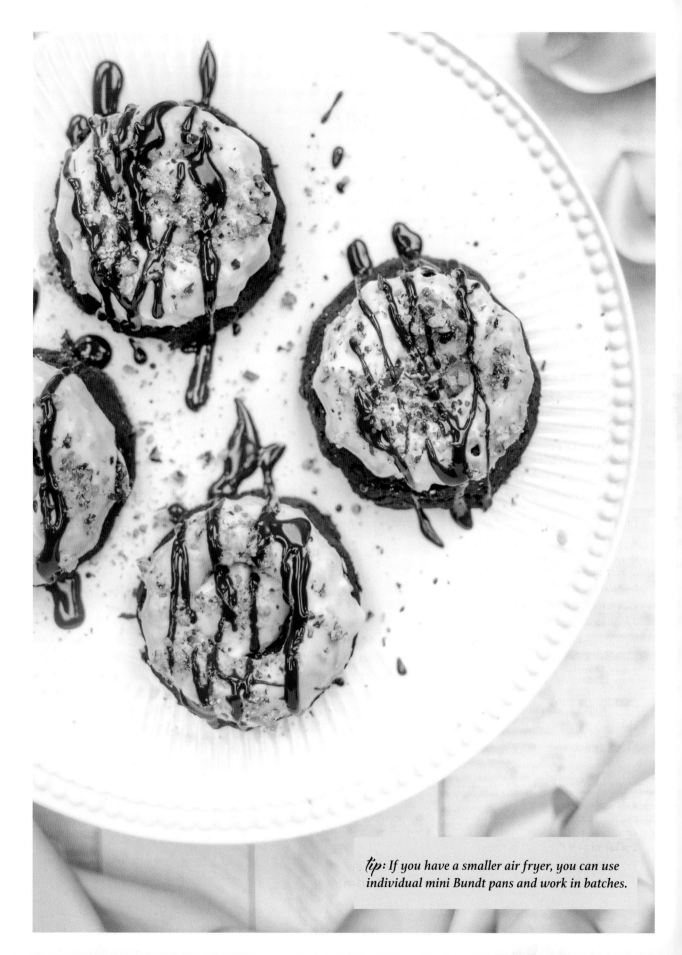

tip: If you have a smaller air fryer, you can use individual mini Bundt pans and work in batches.

Flourless Cream-Filled Mini Cakes

yield: 8 cakes (1 per serving)   *prep time:* 10 minutes   *cook time:* 10 minutes

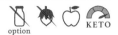

CAKE:

½ cup (1 stick) unsalted butter (or coconut oil for dairy-free)

4 ounces unsweetened chocolate, chopped

¾ cup Swerve confectioners'-style sweetener or equivalent amount of powdered sweetener (see page 18)

3 large eggs

FILLING:

1 (8-ounce) package cream cheese (or Kite Hill brand cream cheese style spread for dairy-free), softened

¼ cup Swerve confectioners'-style sweetener or equivalent amount of powdered or liquid sweetener (see page 18)

FOR GARNISH (OPTIONAL):

Whipped cream

Raspberries

1. Preheat the air fryer to 375°F. Grease eight 4-ounce ramekins.

2. Make the cake batter: Heat the butter and chocolate in a saucepan over low heat, stirring often, until the chocolate is completely melted. Remove from the heat.

3. Add the sweetener and eggs and use a hand mixer on low to combine well. Set aside.

4. Make the cream filling: In a medium-sized bowl, mix together the cream cheese and sweetener until well combined. Taste and add more sweetener if desired.

5. Divide the chocolate mixture among the greased ramekins, filling each one halfway. Place 1 tablespoon of the filling on top of the chocolate mixture in each ramekin.

6. Place the ramekins in the air fryer and cook for 10 minutes, or until the outside is set and the inside is soft and warm. Allow to cool completely, then top with whipped cream, if desired, and garnish with raspberries, if desired.

7. Store without whipped cream in an airtight container in the refrigerator for up to 4 days or in the freezer for up to a month. Serve leftovers chilled or reheat in a preheated 350°F air fryer for 5 minutes, or until heated through.

busy family tip: These taste best right out of the air fryer, but you can store the unbaked cakes in the ramekins in the fridge for up to 5 days and bake one whenever a chocolate craving strikes!

(per serving)   calories **330** | fat **30g** | protein **6g** | total carbs **5g** | fiber **2g**

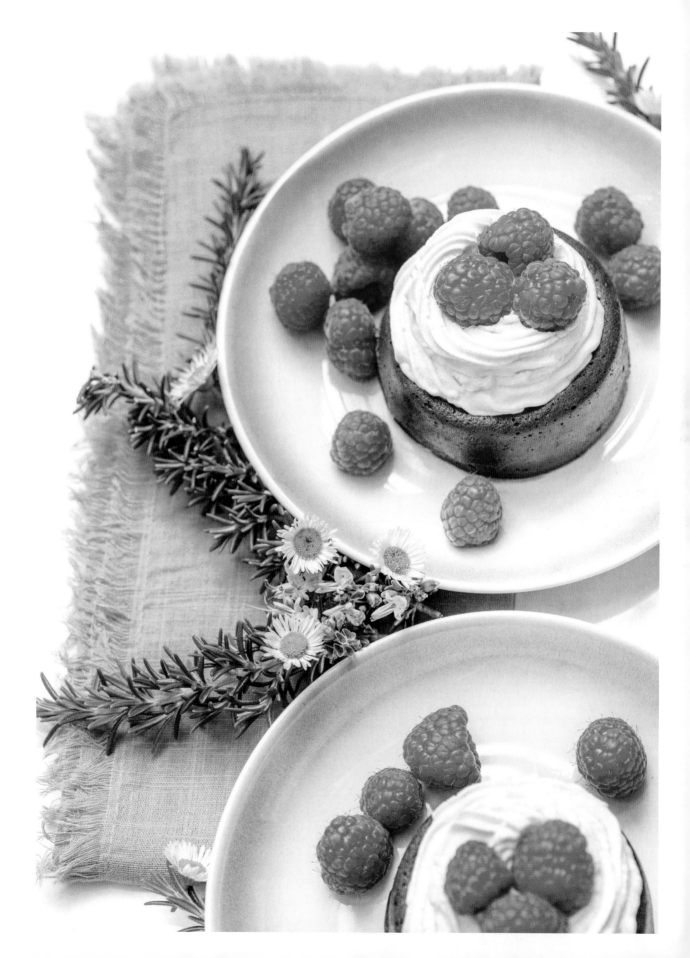

Halle Berries-and-Cream Cobbler

yield: 4 servings   *prep time:* 10 minutes   *cook time:* 25 minutes

KETO

12 ounces cream cheese (1½ cups), softened

1 large egg

¾ cup Swerve confectioners'-style sweetener or equivalent amount of powdered sweetener (see page 18)

½ teaspoon vanilla extract

¼ teaspoon fine sea salt

1 cup sliced fresh raspberries or strawberries

BISCUITS:

3 large egg whites

¾ cup blanched almond flour

1 teaspoon baking powder

2½ tablespoons very cold unsalted butter, cut into pieces (see Tip)

¼ teaspoon fine sea salt

FROSTING:

2 ounces cream cheese (¼ cup), softened

1 tablespoon Swerve confectioners'-style sweetener or equivalent amount of powdered or liquid sweetener (see page 18)

1 tablespoon unsweetened, unflavored almond milk or heavy cream

Fresh raspberries or strawberries, for garnish

1. Preheat the air fryer to 400°F. Grease a 7-inch pie pan.

2. In a large mixing bowl, use a hand mixer to combine the cream cheese, egg, and sweetener until smooth. Stir in the vanilla and salt. Gently fold in the raspberries with a rubber spatula. Pour the mixture into the prepared pan and set aside.

3. Make the biscuits: Place the egg whites in a medium-sized mixing bowl or the bowl of a stand mixer. Using a hand mixer or stand mixer, whip the egg whites until very fluffy and stiff.

4. In a separate medium-sized bowl, combine the almond flour and baking powder. Cut in the butter and add the salt, stirring gently to keep the butter pieces intact.

5. Gently fold the almond flour mixture into the egg whites. Use a large spoon or ice cream scooper to scoop out the dough and form it into a 2-inch-wide biscuit, making sure the butter stays in separate clumps. Place the biscuit on top of the raspberry mixture in the pan. Repeat with remaining dough to make 4 biscuits.

6. Place the pan in the air fryer and cook for 5 minutes, then lower the temperature to 325°F and bake for another 17 to 20 minutes, until the biscuits are golden brown.

7. While the cobbler cooks, make the frosting: Place the cream cheese in a small bowl and stir to break it up. Add the sweetener and stir. Add the almond milk and stir until well combined. If you prefer a thinner frosting, add more almond milk.

8. Remove the cobbler from the air fryer and allow to cool slightly, then drizzle with the frosting. Garnish with fresh raspberries.

9. Store leftovers in an airtight container in the refrigerator for up to 3 days. Reheat the cobbler in a preheated 350°F air fryer for 3 minutes, or until warmed through.

note: I named this recipe in honor of Halle Berry! She eats keto and has all of my cookbooks, and I am very grateful for her support.

tip: The trick to getting the biscuits for this cobbler nice and round with crispy edges is to make sure the butter is very cold—if it's not, the biscuits won't turn out. Also, the air fryer must be preheated.

(per serving)   calories **583** | fat **51g** | protein **16g** | total carbs **10g** | fiber **3g**

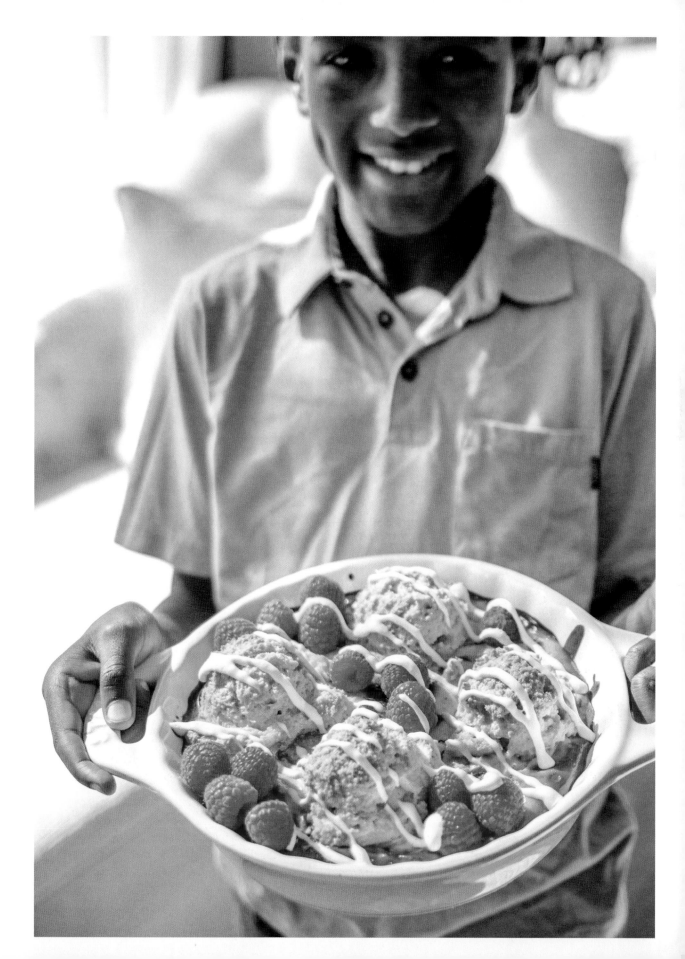

Chocolate Meringue Cookies

yield: 16 cookies (2 per serving)
prep time: 10 minutes, plus 20 minutes to rest *cook time:* 1 hour

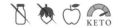

3 large egg whites

¼ teaspoon cream of tartar

¼ cup Swerve confectioners'-style sweetener or equivalent amount of powdered sweetener (see page 18)

2 tablespoons unsweetened cocoa powder

1. Preheat the air fryer to 225°F. Line a 7-inch pie pan or a dish that will fit in your air fryer with parchment paper.

2. In a small bowl, use a hand mixer to beat the egg whites and cream of tartar until soft peaks form. With the mixer on low, slowly sprinkle in the sweetener and mix until it's completely incorporated. Continue to beat with the mixer until stiff peaks form.

3. Add the cocoa powder and gently fold until it's completely incorporated.

4. Spoon the mixture into a piping bag with a ¾-inch tip. (If you don't have a piping bag, snip the corner of a large resealable plastic bag to form a ¾-inch hole.) Pipe sixteen 1-inch meringue cookies onto the lined pie pan, spacing them about ¼ inch apart.

5. Place the pan in the air fryer and cook for 1 hour, until the cookies are crispy on the outside, then turn off the air fryer and let the cookies stand in the air fryer for another 20 minutes before removing and serving.

note: Meringues and humidity do not mix. If your kitchen is very humid, the outside of the meringue won't crisp up.

(per serving)   calories **12** | fat **0.3g** | protein **2g** | total carbs **1g** | fiber **0.3g**

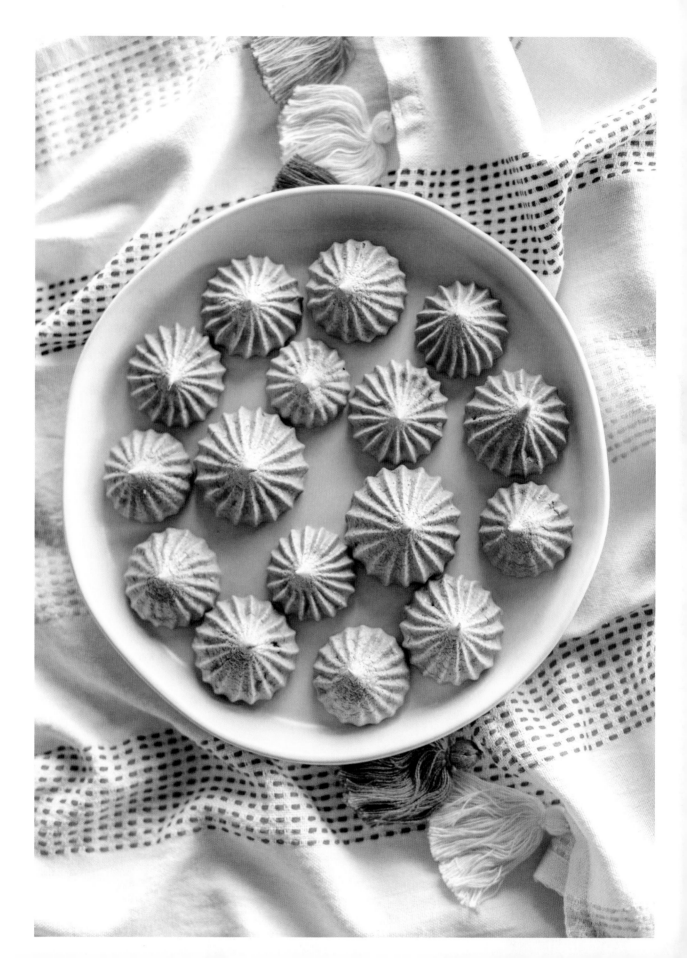

Lemon Poppy Seed Macaroons

yield: 1 dozen cookies *prep time:* 10 minutes *cook time:* 14 minutes

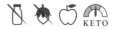

2 large egg whites, room temperature

⅓ cup Swerve confectioners'-style sweetener or equivalent amount of powdered sweetener (see page 18)

2 tablespoons grated lemon zest, plus more for garnish if desired

2 teaspoons poppy seeds

1 teaspoon lemon extract

¼ teaspoon fine sea salt

2 cups unsweetened shredded coconut

LEMON ICING:

¼ cup Swerve confectioners'-style sweetener or equivalent amount of powdered sweetener (see page 18)

1 tablespoon lemon juice

1. Preheat the air fryer to 325°F. Line a 7-inch pie pan or a casserole dish that will fit inside your air fryer with parchment paper.

2. Place the egg whites in a medium-sized bowl and use a hand mixer on high to beat the whites until stiff peaks form. Add the sweetener, lemon zest, poppy seeds, lemon extract, and salt. Mix on low until combined. Gently fold in the coconut with a rubber spatula.

3. Use a 1-inch cookie scoop to place the cookies on the parchment, spacing them about ¼ inch apart. Place the pan in the air fryer and cook for 12 to 14 minutes, until the cookies are golden and a toothpick inserted into the center comes out clean.

4. While the cookies bake, make the lemon icing: Place the sweetener in a small bowl. Add the lemon juice and stir well. If the icing is too thin, add a little more sweetener. If the icing is too thick, add a little more lemon juice.

5. Remove the cookies from the air fryer and allow to cool for about 10 minutes, then drizzle with the icing. Garnish with lemon zest, if desired.

6. Store leftovers in an airtight container in the fridge for up to 5 days or in the freezer for up to a month.

tip: *If your macaroons are flat after baking, most likely one of two things happened:*

- *The whites were underwhipped. This happens a lot. The whites need to be so stiff that you can flip the bowl upside down and they will stay still.*

- *You overmixed when folding in the coconut, which can break down the egg whites. Work quickly but gently and fold only until the batter is mixed well. If the egg whites become runny rather than fluffy, pour the mixture into the prepared pan and make coconut bars—they will still taste delicious!*

(per cookie) calories 71 | fat 7g | protein 1g | total carbs 3g | fiber 2g

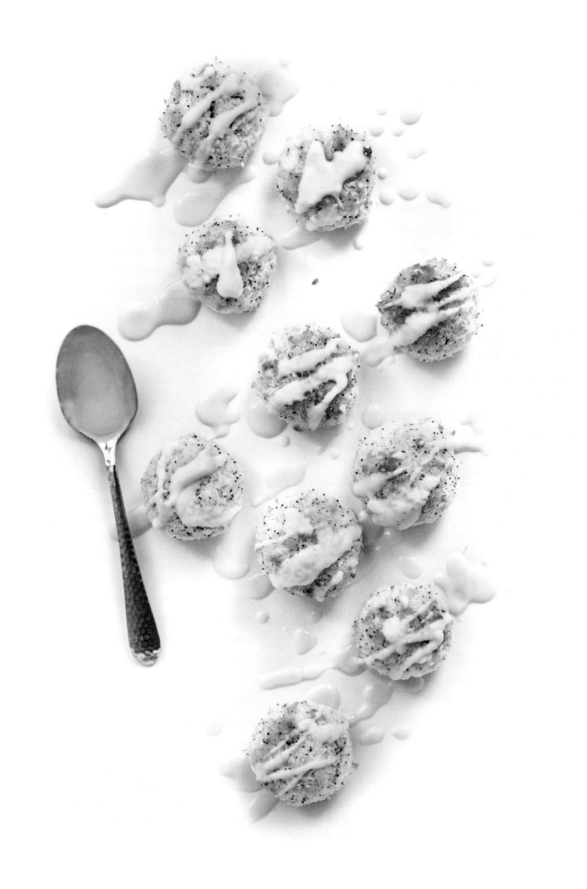

Lemon Curd Pavlova

yield: 4 servings *prep time:* 10 minutes, plus 20 minutes to rest *cook time:* 1 hour

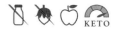

SHELL:

3 large egg whites

¼ teaspoon cream of tartar

¾ cup Swerve confectioners'-style sweetener or equivalent amount of powdered sweetener (see page 18)

1 teaspoon grated lemon zest

1 teaspoon lemon extract

LEMON CURD:

1 cup Swerve confectioners'-style sweetener or equivalent amount of liquid or powdered sweetener (see page 18)

½ cup lemon juice

4 large eggs

½ cup coconut oil

FOR GARNISH (OPTIONAL):

Blueberries

Swerve confectioners'-style sweetener or equivalent amount of powdered sweetener (see page 18)

1. Preheat the air fryer to 275°F. Thoroughly grease a 7-inch pie pan with butter or coconut oil.

2. Make the shell: In a small bowl, use a hand mixer to beat the egg whites and cream of tartar until soft peaks form. With the mixer on low, slowly sprinkle in the sweetener and mix until it's completely incorporated.

3. Add the lemon zest and lemon extract and continue to beat with the hand mixer until stiff peaks form.

4. Spoon the mixture into the greased pie pan, then smooth it across the bottom, up the sides, and onto the rim to form a shell. Cook for 1 hour, then turn off the air fryer and let the shell stand in the air fryer for 20 minutes. (The shell can be made up to 3 days ahead and stored in an airtight container in the refrigerator, if desired.)

5. While the shell bakes, make the lemon curd: In a medium-sized heavy-bottomed saucepan, whisk together the sweetener, lemon juice, and eggs. Add the coconut oil and place the pan on the stovetop over medium heat. Once the oil is melted, whisk constantly until the mixture thickens and thickly coats the back of a spoon, about 10 minutes. Do not allow the mixture to come to a boil.

6. Pour the lemon curd mixture through a fine-mesh strainer into a medium-sized bowl. Place the bowl inside a larger bowl filled with ice water and whisk occasionally until the curd is completely cool, about 15 minutes.

7. Place the lemon curd on top of the shell and garnish with blueberries and powdered sweetener, if desired. Store leftovers in the refrigerator for up to 4 days.

tip: *Meringues and humidity do not mix. If your kitchen is very humid, the outside of the meringue won't crisp up.*

(per serving) calories **332** | fat **33g** | protein **9g** | total carbs **4g** | fiber **1g**

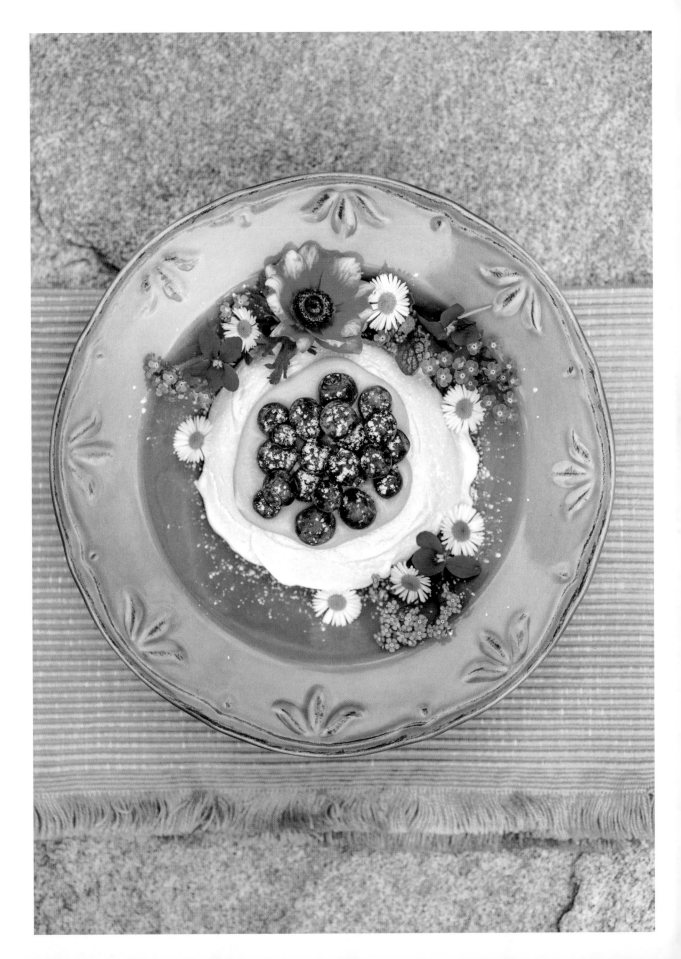

Acknowledgments

There are many special people that I need to thank for making this book possible and beautiful!

I have intense gratitude to the whole Victory Belt team. I never thought I would have such amazing support and kindness from everyone at Victory Belt. I am grateful for all of your hard work and dedication to always make my books stunning!

To my dear Erin, my editor, this book is amazing because of the care and time you have put into this! I'm thankful for the care and attention to detail you put into this book. I know that there were long hours put into *Keto Air Fryer,* and I am very grateful for you!

Susan, I am grateful for your passion and for how magnificently you help to publicize my books, and for traveling with me to New York to help me on my television segment. I get a smile on my face whenever I receive an email from you. Your happiness shines through!

Lance, I can't thank you enough for helping with all of my questions and creating amazingly beautiful images for promoting this lovely book.

Erich, your praise and fun outlook made this journey extraordinary and totally worth the hard work and long days of writing, editing, cooking, and photographing! I appreciate your caring phone calls just to check in on me and make sure everything was going smoothly.

I also want to thank my recipe testers! Wendy (who has a type 1 diabetes and sends her readings to me after testing my recipes), Erin, Jodi, and Leisa are my beloved recipe testers and have spent numerous hours trying my recipes and making sure they taste amazing. Their time and hard work were essential to make the tasty dishes in this cookbook. And a special thank-you to Jennifer, who is also one of my keto coaches. She not only tested recipes for this book, but she also took many of the photos!

Bill and Hayley, I am honored to have your photo for the cover for this book. I've always been a big fan of your photos and cookbooks. My first Victory Belt cookbook was your book *Gather.* I was in love with your artistry from the beginning. I thought I was the only one who loved my job so much that I always get up before the sun, even on Sunday mornings, but you shot the cover photo early on a Sunday morning. Thank you so much for your dedication and lovely cover photos!

I am grateful to my love and best friend, Craig, who never complains even though I often mess up the kitchen as soon as he cleans it. He has also been a huge part of this book by picking up all the groceries, testing recipes, and adding the detailed nutritional information for all the recipes.

I am grateful for my boys, Micah and Kai, who love to help me in the kitchen. Even though it takes twice as long to get dinner on the table when they help me, it is totally worth it. When we had to put our adoption on hold, I was completely devastated, but I remember my mom telling me that my children just weren't born yet. I cry as I write this because she was totally right. These two boys were meant for me!

I also want to express my gratitude to you, the reader! I can't thank you enough for all your love and support through my journey!

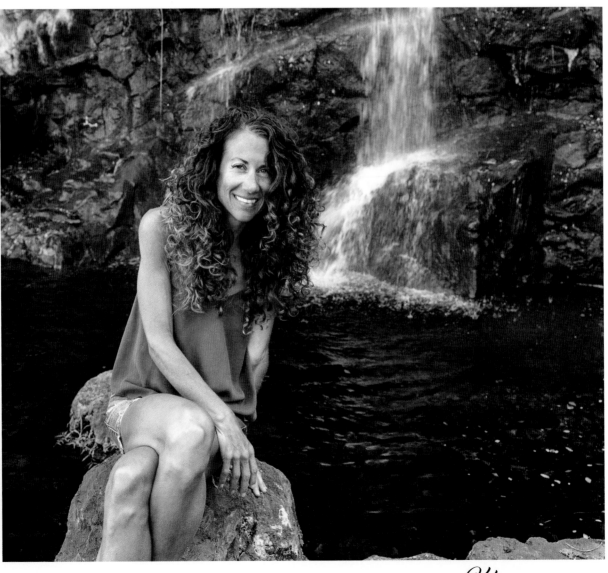

Allergen Index

Recipe	Page	🥛	🥑	🌰	🍎	KETO
Bacon-and-Eggs Avocado	22	✓		✓		L
Double-Dipped Mini Cinnamon Biscuits	24				✓	L
Meritage Eggs	26	O		✓	✓	H
Breakfast Pizza	28	O		O	O	H
Denver Omelet	30	O			O	H
Easy Bacon	32	✓	✓	✓		H
Valerie's Breakfast Sammies	34	O				H
Gyro Breakfast Patties with Tzatziki	36		✓	✓		H
The Best Keto Quiche	38				O	M
Easy Mexican Shakshuka	40	✓		✓	✓	L
Green Eggs and Ham	42	O		✓		L
Everything Bagels	44				✓	L
Keto Danish	46	O		O	✓	H
French Toast Pavlova	48			✓	✓	H
Breakfast Cobbler	50					M
Buffalo Cauliflower	54		✓	✓	✓	L
Ranch Kale Chips	56	✓	✓	✓	✓	L
Crispy Nacho Avocado Fries	58	✓		✓	O	L
Bacon-Wrapped Pickle Poppers	60		✓	✓		H
Bourbon Chicken Wings	62	✓	✓	✓		H
Doro Wat Wings	64	✓	O	✓		H
Salt and Vinegar Pork Belly Chips	66	✓	✓	✓		H
Crispy Prosciutto-Wrapped Onion Rings	68	O	✓	✓		H
Bacon-Wrapped Asparagus	70	O	✓	✓		M
Reuben Egg Rolls	72			✓		H
Mozzarella Sticks	74				✓	M
Crispy Calamari Rings	76	O		✓		L
Bloomin' Onion	78	O		✓	✓	L
Prosciutto-Wrapped Guacamole Rings	80	✓	✓	✓		L
Prosciutto Pierogi	82	O	✓	✓		H
Keto Tots	86	O		✓	✓	M
Loaded Bacon-Wrapped Keto Tots	88			✓		M
Tomatoes Provençal	90		✓	✓	✓	L
Burrata-Stuffed Tomatoes	92		✓	✓	✓	M
Crispy Brussels Sprouts	93	O	✓	✓	✓	L
Caramelized Broccoli	94	O	O	✓	✓	L
Perfect Zoodles	95	✓	✓	✓	✓	L
Marinated Turmeric Cauliflower Steaks	96	O	✓	✓	✓	L

Recipe	Page	🥛	🥑	🍓	🍎	KETO
Caramelized Ranch Cauliflower	97	✓	✓	✓	✓	L
Fried Cauliflower Rice	98	✓	✓	✓	O	L
Garlic Thyme Mushrooms	99	O	✓	✓	✓	M
Sweet Fauxtato Casserole	100	O			✓	L
Spinach Artichoke Tart	102				✓	L
Crunchy-Top Personal Mac 'n' Cheese	104		✓	✓		M
Parmesan Flan	106			✓	O	H
Garlic Butter Breadsticks	108				✓	M
Bruschetta	110	O			✓	L
Savory Beefy Poppers	114	O	✓	✓		H
Swedish Meatloaf	116		O	✓		H
Carne Asada	118	✓	✓	✓		M
Salisbury Steak with Mushroom Onion Gravy	120	O	✓	✓		M
Fajita Meatball Lettuce Wraps	122	✓		✓		H
Reuben Fritters	124		O	✓		H
Greek Stuffed Tenderloin	126		✓	✓		H
Herb-Crusted Lamb Chops	128	O		✓		H
Black 'n' Blue Burgers	130	O				H
Mojito Lamb Chops	132	✓	✓	✓		H
Mushroom and Swiss Burgers	134	O	✓	✓		H
Deconstructed Chicago Dogs	138	✓	✓	✓		H
Pork Milanese	140	O		✓		H
Italian Sausages with Peppers and Onions	142	✓	✓	✓		H
Scotch Eggs	144	✓		✓		H
Mama Maria's Savory Sausage Cobbler	146					M
Pork Tenderloin with Avocado Lime Sauce	148	O	✓	✓		H
Five-Spice Pork Belly	150	✓	✓	✓		H
BBQ Riblets	152	✓	✓	✓		H
Dry Rub Baby Back Ribs	154	✓	✓	✓		H
Bacon-Wrapped Stuffed Pork Chops	156	O	✓	✓		H
Chicken Kiev	160	O		✓		H
Chicken Cordon Bleu Meatballs	162			✓		H
Buffalo Chicken Drumsticks	164		✓	✓		H
Sesame Turkey Balls in Lettuce Cups	166	✓		✓		H
Porchetta-Style Chicken Breasts	168	✓	✓	✓		H
Easy Thanksgiving Turkey Breast	170		✓	✓		H
Chicken Paillard	172			✓		H
General Tso's Chicken	174	✓	✓	✓		H
Chicken Strips with Satay Sauce	176	✓	✓	O		H
Bacon Lovers' Stuffed Chicken	178	O	✓	✓		H

Recipe	Page	🍼	🥑	🌿	🍎	KETO
Chicken Pesto Parmigiana	180			O		H
Crispy Taco Chicken	182	O		✓		H
Thai Tacos with Peanut Sauce	184	✓	✓			M
Shrimp Scampi	188	O	✓	✓		H
Simple Scallops	190	✓	✓	✓		H
Tuna Melt Croquettes	192			✓		H
Coconut Shrimp with Spicy Mayo	194	✓		✓		H
Crispy Crab Rangoon Patties with Sweet 'n' Sour Sauce	196			✓		H
Pecan-Crusted Catfish	198	✓	✓			H
Friday Night Fish Fry	200	O		✓		H
Parmesan-Crusted Shrimp over Pesto Zoodles	202			O		H
Asian Marinated Salmon	204	✓	✓	✓		H
BLT Crab Cakes	206	O		✓		H
Mouthwatering Cod over Creamy Leek Noodles	208			✓		H
Spicy Popcorn Shrimp	210			✓		H
Breaded Shrimp Tacos	212			✓		H
Ham 'n' Cheese Hand Pies	216					H
Cheeseburger Meatballs	218			✓		H
Keto Turtles	220	✓	✓	✓		H
No-Corn Dogs	222					H
Italian Dunkers	224	✓		✓		H
Hot Dog Buns	226	✓			✓	L
BLT Sushi	228	✓		✓		H
Popcorn Chicken	230			✓		H
Ham 'n' Cheese Ravioli	232			✓		H
Chicken Patties	234	O		✓		H
Little French Fudge Cakes	238	O			✓	L
Flourless Cream-Filled Mini Cakes	240	O		✓	✓	H
Halle Berries-and-Cream Cobbler	242				✓	L
Chocolate Meringue Cookies	244	✓		✓	✓	H
Lemon Poppy Seed Macaroons	246	✓		✓	✓	M
Lemon Curd Pavlova	248	✓		✓	✓	H

Recipe Index

Breakfast

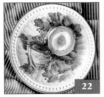
Bacon-and-Eggs Avocado
22

Double-Dipped Mini Cinnamon Biscuits
24

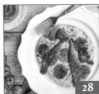
Meritage Eggs
26

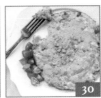
Breakfast Pizza
28

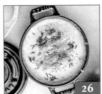
Denver Omelet
30

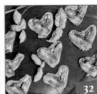
Easy Bacon
32

Valerie's Breakfast Sammies
34

Gyro Breakfast Patties with Tzatziki
36

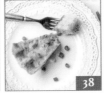
The Best Keto Quiche
38

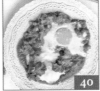
Easy Mexican Shakshuka
40

Green Eggs and Ham
42

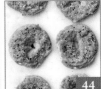
Everything Bagels
44

Keto Danish
46

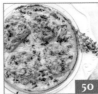
French Toast Pavlova
48

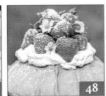
Breakfast Cobbler
50

Appetizers

 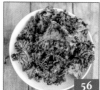   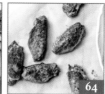 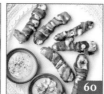

Buffalo Cauliflower 54 **Ranch Kale Chips** 56 **Crispy Nacho Avocado Fries** 58 **Bacon-Wrapped Pickle Poppers** 60 **Bourbon Chicken Wings** 62 **Doro Wat Wings** 64

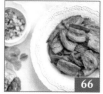   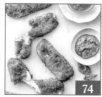 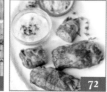 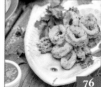

Salt and Vinegar Pork Belly Chips 66 **Crispy Prosciutto-Wrapped Onion Rings** 68 **Bacon-Wrapped Asparagus** 70 **Reuben Egg Rolls** 72 **Mozzarella Sticks** 74 **Crispy Calamari Rings** 76

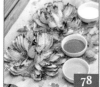 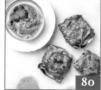

Bloomin' Onion 78 **Prosciutto-Wrapped Guacamole Rings** 80 **Prosciutto Pierogi** 82

Sides and Vegetarian

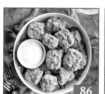 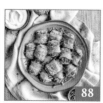 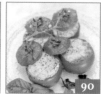 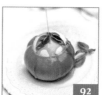 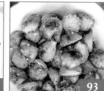 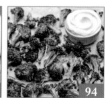

Keto Tots 86 **Loaded Bacon-Wrapped Keto Tots** 88 **Tomatoes Provençal** 90 **Burrata-Stuffed Tomatoes** 92 **Crispy Brussels Sprouts** 93 **Caramelized Broccoli** 94

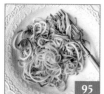 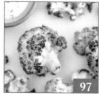 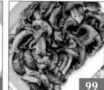

Perfect Zoodles 95 **Marinated Turmeric Cauliflower Steaks** 96 **Caramelized Ranch Cauliflower** 97 **Fried Cauliflower Rice** 98 **Garlic Thyme Mushrooms** 99 **Sweet Fauxtato Casserole** 100

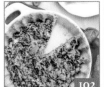
Spinach Artichoke
Tart 102

Crunchy-Top
Personal
Mac 'n' Cheese 104

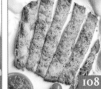
Parmesan Flan 106

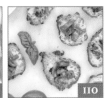
Garlic Butter
Breadsticks 108

Bruschetta 110

Beef and Lamb

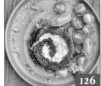
Savory Beefy
Poppers 114

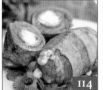
Swedish Meatloaf 116

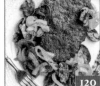
Carne Asada 118

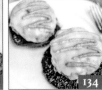
Salisbury Steak with
Mushroom Onion
Gravy 120

Fajita Meatball
Lettuce Wraps 122

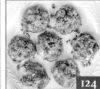
Reuben Fritters 124

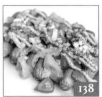
Greek Stuffed
Tenderloin 126

Herb-Crusted
Lamb Chops 128

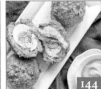
Black 'n' Blue
Burgers 130

Mojito Lamb Chops 132

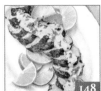
Mushroom and
Swiss Burgers 134

Pork

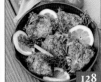
Deconstructed
Chicago Dogs 138

Pork Milanese 140

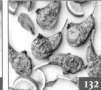
Italian Sausages
with Peppers and
Onions 142

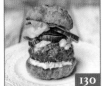
Scotch Eggs 144

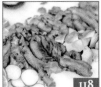
Mama Maria's
Savory Sausage
Cobbler 146

Pork Tenderloin
with Avocado Lime
Sauce 148

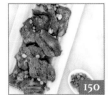
Five-Spice Pork Belly 150

BBQ Riblets 152

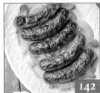
Dry Rub
Baby Back Ribs 154

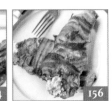
Bacon-Wrapped
Stuffed Pork Chops 156

Poultry

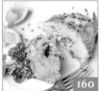
Chicken Kiev
160

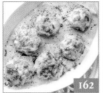
Chicken Cordon
Bleu Meatballs
162

Buffalo Chicken
Drumsticks
164

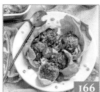
Sesame Turkey Balls
in Lettuce Cups
166

Porchetta-Style
Chicken Breasts
168

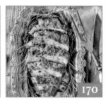
Easy Thanksgiving
Turkey Breast
170

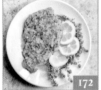
Chicken Paillard
172

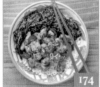
General Tso's
Chicken
174

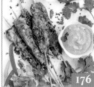
Chicken Strips with
Satay Sauce
176

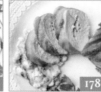
Bacon Lovers'
Stuffed Chicken
178

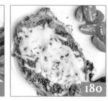
Chicken Pesto
Parmigiana
180

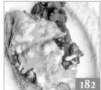
Crispy Taco Chicken
182

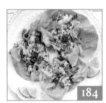
Thai Tacos with
Peanut Sauce
184

Fish and Seafood

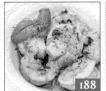
Shrimp Scampi

Simple Scallops

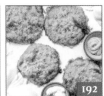
Tuna Melt
Croquettes

Coconut Shrimp
with Spicy Mayo

Crispy Crab Rangoon
Patties with
Sweet 'n' Sour Sauce

Pecan-Crusted
Catfish

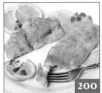
Friday Night
Fish Fry

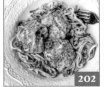
Parmesan-Crusted
Shrimp over
Pesto Zoodles

Asian Marinated
Salmon

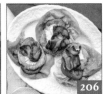
BLT Crab Cakes

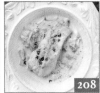
Mouthwatering Cod
over Creamy
Leek Noodles

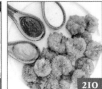
Spicy Popcorn
Shrimp

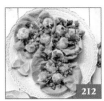
Breaded Shrimp
Tacos

Kid Classics

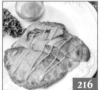
216
Ham 'n' Cheese
Hand Pies

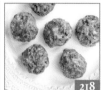
218
Cheeseburger
Meatballs

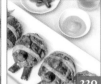
220
Keto Turtles

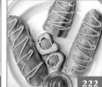
222
No-Corn Dogs

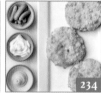
224
Italian Dunkers

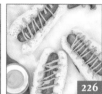
226
Hot Dog Buns

228
BLT Sushi

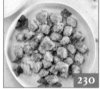
230
Popcorn Chicken

232
Ham 'n' Cheese
Ravioli

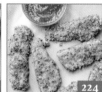
234
Chicken Patties

Sweet Endings

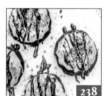
238
Little French Fudge
Cakes

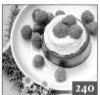
240
Flourless Cream-
Filled Mini Cakes

242
Halle Berries-and-
Cream Cobbler

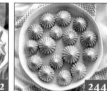
244
Chocolate Meringue
Cookies

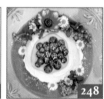
246
Lemon Poppy Seed
Macaroons

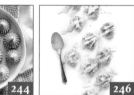
248
Lemon Curd Pavlova

General Index